THE WAISTLINE PLAN

1   3   4   5   6   7   8   9   10   11   12   13

hamlyn

THE WAISTLINE PLAN
BEAT MIDDLE-AGE SPREAD IN JUST 6 WEEKS!

14 15 16 17 18 19 20 21 22 23 24 25 26

Sally Lewis

Notes

It is advisable to check with your doctor before embarking on any exercise programme. This book is not intended as a substitute for personal medical advice. The reader should consult a doctor in all matters relating to health and particularly in respect of any symptoms that may require diagnosis or medical attention. While the advice and information are believed to be accurate and true at the time of going to press, neither the author nor the publisher can accept any legal responsibility or liability for errors or omissions that may be made.

Both metric and imperial measurements have been given in all recipes. Use one set of measurements only, and not a mixture of both.

Standard level spoon measurements are used in all recipes.
1 tablespoon = one 15 ml spoon
1 teaspoon = one 5 ml spoon

Ovens should be preheated to the specified temperature – if using a fan-assisted oven, follow the manufacturer's instructions for adjusting the time and the temperature.

Fresh herbs should be used unless otherwise stated.

Medium eggs should be used unless otherwise stated.

The Department of Health advises that eggs should not be consumed raw. This book contains some dishes made with raw or lightly cooked eggs. It is prudent for vulnerable people such as pregnant and nursing mothers, invalids, the elderly, babies and young children to avoid uncooked or lightly cooked dishes made with eggs. Once prepared, these dishes should be kept refrigerated and used promptly.

This book includes dishes made with nuts and nut derivatives. It is advisable for those with known allergic reactions to nuts and nut derivatives and those who may be potentially vulnerable to these allergies, such as pregnant and nursing mothers, invalids, the elderly, babies and children, to avoid dishes made with nuts and nut oils. It is also prudent to check the labels of pre-prepared ingredients for the possible inclusion of nut derivatives.

First published in Great Britain in 2007 by Hamlyn,
a division of Octopus Publishing Group Ltd
2–4 Heron Quays, London E14 4JP

Copyright © Octopus Publishing Group Ltd 2007

Distributed in the United States and Canada by Sterling Publishing Co., Inc., 387 Park Avenue South, New York, NY 10016–8810

ISBN-13: 978-0-600-61562-0
ISBN-10: 0-600-61562-6

A CIP catalogue record for this book is available from the British Library

Printed and bound in China

10 9 8 7 6 5 4 3 2 1

CONTENTS

INTRODUCTION

Middle-age spread is something that affects us all. It's an age-related, hormonal condition that has serious health implications. Research shows that women especially are prone to rapid weight gain in middle age, a time when hormonal changes alter metabolism and increase appetite by up to 67 per cent. However, men, too, are prone to midriff spread from their thirties onwards, and the health implications of the condition are no less serious for them.

THE BATTLE OF THE BULGE

The good news is that you can fight back against middle-age weight gain – and this book will show you how. The Waistline Plan is all about making small changes in the way you eat and exercise and, most importantly, in the

way you understand your body. Getting to know your nutritional needs, raising your metabolism, controlling your blood sugar levels, balancing your hormones and spending a little time on exercise will help you to control the spread of excess weight around your middle, no matter what your age. By following the delicious menu plan and some simple fitness routines for just 6 weeks you can lose 6 kg (14 lb); you will look and feel slimmer, fitter and younger. Once you have achieved your target weight, you can use the Diet Maintenance Plan (see page 27) to keep the weight off for good.

The Waistline Diet Plan

The easy-to-follow 42-day menu plan includes tasty recipes, nutritional advice, ideas for healthy snacks and tips to keep you motivated. The food options are flexible and filling, with alternatives for breakfast, lunch and dinner, plus two nutritious snacks per day – so you won't even notice that you're on a diet and you and your family certainly won't get bored!

The Waistline Exercise Plan

You don't have to spend hours exercising to make a difference. Just 10 minutes of toning exercises, repeated 3 times a day, 5 days a week, combined with a single weekly session of aerobic exercise, will have a fantastic impact on your health and fitness. With only minor adjustments to your usual schedule, you'll be able to lose that excess weight and tone up your body. All the toning exercises are specifically designed to target the areas where middle-age spread is common – around the stomach, waist, hips, thighs and buttocks.

WHAT'S SPECIAL ABOUT THE PLAN?

The Waistline Plan really works, because it's not based on any faddish or very demanding regimes. It simply combats the nutritional, medical and lifestyle causes of middle-age spread with a simple approach to healthy eating and exercise that can be adopted by anyone.

- Unlike other diets, the Waistline Diet Plan doesn't deprive you of food. It actively encourages you to eat — and shows you how to make the right food choices.
- Regular, healthy meals and snacks each day will help to stabilize your blood sugar levels and eliminate those unhealthy cravings.
- The menus include foods to boost your metabolism and balance your hormones, both of which can have a huge effect in helping you to keep weight off your middle.
- You won't be cutting out any important food groups, but you will reduce your intake of sugar and salt. You do eat fats — but only those that are good for you.
- There is no need to calorie count.
- The whole family will enjoy the recipes, so there is no need to cook different meals.
- The Waistline Exercise Plan is very flexible and specially designed to fit into busy lives. Workouts can be as short as 10 minutes, but you can easily make them longer.
- Toning and aerobic exercise together produce great results, by burning fat and firming up your body.

WHY MOST DIETS DON'T WORK

Diets often fail because people get bored with them or because they limit food intake so excessively that dieters find themselves hungry and craving certain foods — and just end up reaching for those biscuits or chocolates. There are also nutritional reasons why 'yo-yo' dieters so often fail. Depriving the body of food simply places it in a fasting state, making it hang on to the fat you are trying to shift. Starvation causes the metabolism to slow down, so there is a danger of putting on weight as soon as you eat normally. What's more, when the body's intake of food is restricted it becomes stressed. Stress causes blood sugar levels to fluctuate, creating excess glucose with nowhere to go except to make more fat (see page 12).

This book will help you to understand the nutritional needs of your body. You'll find out what makes your hormones swing into action and cause weight gain, how ageing changes your body and how stress can have a dangerous effect on your wellbeing. This information will enable you to manage the lifestyle changes you are about to make through the Waistline Plan.

WHY SIZE MATTERS

Middle-age spread is part of a recognized medical condition known as the somatopause. It can have serious consequences, affecting your energy, memory, mood and libido, as well as your muscle and bone density, skin quality and cholesterol levels, and increasing the risk of disease. You may only be in your mid-thirties, but your body will look and act older than your age. By showing you how to fight middle-age spread, the Waistline Plan will help to restore your vitality and give you the chance of leading a longer, healthier life.

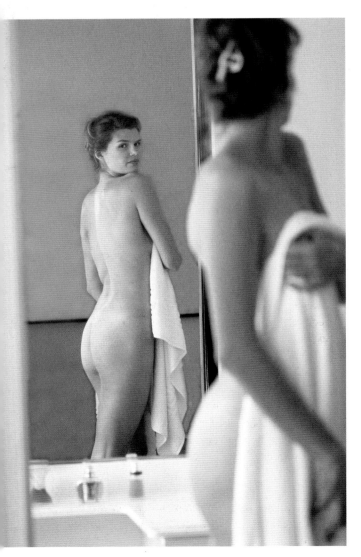

Heart disease and stroke

Heart disease is one of the biggest causes of disability and death in the West. People who eat a typical Western diet tend to accumulate fatty deposits on their artery walls, which in turn lead to arteriosclerosis – narrowing and hardening of the arteries. This can cause angina, severe chest pain, stroke and heart attack. Overweight people are also more likely to suffer from hypertension (raised blood pressure), increasing their risk of heart disease and stroke.

If you are overweight, reducing your weight by 10 per cent can decrease your risk of developing heart disease, reduce your blood pressure, and also lower the levels of 'bad' low-density lipoprotein (LDL) cholesterol and triglycerides (which are also fats) in your blood.

Diabetes

Statistically, overweight people – those with a Body Mass Index (BMI) of 25 or over (see page 10) – are twice as likely to develop Type 2 diabetes as people who are not overweight. Non insulin-dependent diabetes mellitus (Type 2 diabetes) is the most common type of diabetes in the West. It is a long-term condition, in which the body is unable to regulate the amount of glucose (sugar) in the blood properly. It occurs when the body no longer responds adequately to the natural hormone insulin (see page 12) or when the production of insulin is too low.

The good news is that Type 2 diabetes can usually be controlled through diet, exercise and medication. If poorly controlled, it increases the risk of heart disease, strokes, nerve damage and blindness. People who are an 'apple shape' – with lots of fat around the abdomen – are at greater risk of developing this type of diabetes.

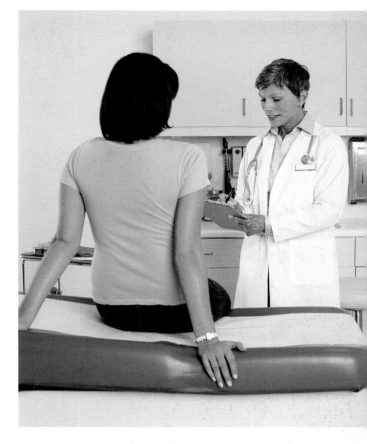

Osteoarthritis

This is a common and painful joint disorder that most often affects the joints in the knees, hips and lower back. Being overweight appears to increase the risk of osteoarthritis, by placing extra pressure on the joints and wearing away the cartilage – the tissue that cushions the joints and normally protects them.

Cancer

Several types of cancer are associated with obesity. In women, these include cancer of the uterus, gallbladder, cervix, ovary, breast and colon. Overweight men are at greater risk of developing cancer of the colon, rectum and prostate.

For some types of cancer, such as colon or breast, it is not clear whether the increased risk is due to the extra weight or to a high-fat and high-calorie diet – this, of course, being strongly associated with weight problems.

Gallbladder disease

Gallbladder disease is most often caused by gallstones. These are more common in people who are overweight, and the risk of the disease increases as weight increases. It is thought that the condition is caused by changes in the way the body handles fat and cholesterol, leading to an over-saturation of bile.

Sleep apnoea

This is a serious condition that is closely associated with being overweight. It can cause a person to stop breathing for short periods during sleep and to snore heavily. As a further consequence, there may be daytime sleepiness and, in extreme cases, the onset of symptoms of heart failure. The risk of sleep apnoea increases with higher body weights.

Fatigue

Being overweight makes you tired, not just because of the extra weight you are carrying but also due to changes in hormone production as the body gradually becomes insulin resistant (see pages 12–13). As a consequence, you will become increasingly tired, and in the long run you may develop Type 2 diabetes.

Back pain

Any excess weight places extra strain on your body, and if you are carrying excess weight around your middle then it is more than likely that your stomach muscles are not being exercised and are weak. Strong stomach muscles support the back and help prevent back pain.

Infertility

Being overweight reduces a woman's chances of becoming pregnant, as it affects hormone production and ovulation.

UNDERSTANDING WEIGHT AND FAT

Two methods can be used to identify whether you are overweight. Body Mass Index (BMI) is used internationally as a way of determining whether your weight is putting your health at risk. BMI considers weight and height and it is best used in conjunction with the waist-to-hip ratio (WHR) measurement, which calculates your percentage of body fat. Some professionals consider your WHR to be more accurate for assessing health risks, as it measures abdominal fat – the fat most associated with health problems.

BODY MASS INDEX

There are two ways of finding out if you are the right weight for your height. Refer to the weight-height chart (right) to see if you are underweight, normal weight, overweight, obese or severely obese. If your weight is at the lower end of the normal range, try to maintain it and don't be tempted to aim for the underweight category.

Calculating your BMI

You can also use this method to calculate your BMI.

1 Measure your height in metres and multiply this figure by itself.
2 Measure your weight in kilograms.
3 Divide the weight by the height squared. For example, the BMI for someone who weighs 65 kg (10 stone) and is 1.7 m (5 ft 7 in) tall is: 65 divided by (1.7 x 1.7) = 22.5. This weight would be within the normal range.

What does it mean?

below 18.5   underweight
18.5–25   normal weight
25–30   overweight
30–35   obese
above 35   severely obese

The range from 18.5 to 25 is quite wide, as 'normal' weight-for-height covers men and women and people of different shapes and body composition. A man usually has a higher BMI than a woman of the same height, as men tend to have more muscle (muscle weighs more than fat). A slim, muscular woman will have a higher BMI than a slim, not very muscular woman of the same height.

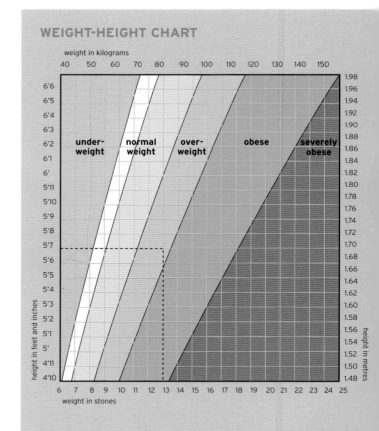

WEIGHT-HEIGHT CHART

The example shown by the dotted line describes the BMI of someone who is 1.7 m (5 ft 7 in) tall and weighs 82 kg (13 stone). This gives a BMI in the top end of the overweight category.

WAIST-TO-HIP RATIO

The waist-to-hip ratio (WHR) is used to determine how much body fat you are carrying. This measurement is thought to be a more reliable guide to your risk of health problems than the BMI calculation, as it is possible to have a high BMI and a normal waist measurement if, for example, you are a fit, lean, muscular man.

You can work out your WHR by dividing your waist measurement by your hip measurement. For women, the ratio should not be over 0.85; for men, it should not be over 0.90. The higher the number above these values, the greater the risk of heart disease and other problems.

Calculating your WHR

1 Measure your waist circumference at the narrowest part. Slowly breathe out – don't hold in your stomach. Do not pull the tape too tight.
2 Measure your hip circumference at the widest part.
3 Divide your waist measurement by your hip measurement. For example, the WHR of a woman with a waist measuring 89 cm (35 in) and hips measuring 104 cm (41 in) is: 89 (35) divided by 104 (41) = 0.85. This is at the top end of the normal range.

WAIST CIRCUMFERENCE

In addition to the BMI and WHR calculations, you can use your waist circumference measurement to evaluate whether you are at risk of obesity complications and mortality. In women, a waist circumference above 89 cm (35 in) confers increased risk. In men, the risks begin to rise at a measurement of 102 cm (40 in).

ALL ABOUT BODY FAT

Normal levels of fat are not a problem for the body. Fat is an energy reservoir, laid down when food is plentiful and converted back to energy when needed. However, when too much of the wrong kind of food is consumed, and calorie intake is higher than calorie expenditure, weight is accumulated. Eventually, this can lead to obesity.

Fat may be subcutaneous or visceral. Subcutaneous fat lies just under the skin, while visceral fat is stored deep inside the body. It is the visceral fat in the midriff section of the body (sometimes known as intra-abdominal fat) and its proximity to the portal vein – a major vessel that feeds the liver – that increase the risk of disease. Visceral fat releases substances that may flow directly into the liver and set off a chain of events that can lead to insulin resistance and the suppression of leptin, a hormone-like substance that tells the brain when you are full (see pages 12–13).

Most fat is stored under the skin, but, as well as visceral fat, there is also some on top of the kidneys and inside the liver and muscles. Other body parts that gather fat depend on gender: men are prone to storing fat on the chest, middle and buttocks (apple shape), while women accumulate fat on the breasts, waist, hips, buttocks and thighs (pear shape). Following the drop in oestrogen levels after the menopause, women too begin to accumulate fat around the middle.

CAUSES OF MIDDLE-AGE SPREAD

While genetics play a role in the accumulation of middle-age spread, it doesn't have to be a fact of life. From lack of exercise and unbalanced hormones to stress and pollutants, there are many reasons why you may gain weight around your abdomen and hips as you get older. The Waistline Plan tackles middle-age spread by addressing its underlying causes, whether through exercise or by foods that balance hormones and boost the metabolism (see pages 17–19).

Hormones

The hormones directly related to appetite include leptin, insulin and ghrelin. When working in harmony they help to maintain a healthy body weight, but factors including stress, lifestyle and processed foods can knock them off balance and result in weight gain. A healthy diet that includes foods which help to balance your hormones can help you to lose weight (see pages 17–18).

- **Leptin** This hormone suppresses appetite. Produced by fatty tissues, it travels to the hypothalamus, the brain's appetite centre, where it induces satiation. At the same time, it stimulates the nervous system, urging the body to increase its metabolism. When leptin levels in the blood and brain drop, the signal to eat takes over again.

- **Ghrelin** This recently discovered hunger hormone both stimulates the desire to eat and controls the feeling of hunger. The levels of ghrelin fall when you eat, but this is affected by the type of food: carbohydrates have the greatest effect and fat the smallest. You are much more likely to feel hungrier, quicker, after eating fatty food than a carbohydrate-rich meal.

- **Insulin** Produced by the pancreas, this hormone regulates carbohydrate metabolism. Secretion of insulin increases rapidly after eating. Most body cells have insulin receptors that bind circulating insulin, allowing glucose (sugar) to be absorbed from the bloodstream into cells. However, when you are overweight, high levels of uncontrolled insulin circulate within your body. Excess insulin may also be released if blood sugar increases constantly as a reaction to stress (see below). If the glucose is not used up it is stored as fat and, furthermore, the continual production of insulin eventually makes the body insulin resistant. It will then be difficult for you to lose weight, and you will also increase your chances of developing Type 2 diabetes (see page 8).

Stress

One of the biggest contributors to increasing abdominal fat, stress affects the adrenal glands. These are located near the kidneys and produce the hormones cortisol and adrenalin, releasing them into the bloodstream. When healthy, the adrenals increase heart rate and blood pressure, release energy stores for immediate use, slow digestion and sharpen the senses. Under continual stress, however, they remain on constant alert.

DID YOU KNOW?

- Natural sunlight is an appetite suppressant, as it helps to regulate hormones associated with hunger. You typically eat less when the weather is warm and sunny.

- During the perimenopause and menopause, erratic hormone fluctuations can cause rapid weight gain and changes in body shape.

- Women's bodies are more prone to hormonal imbalance than men's. Women gain weight, lose weight and maintain weight at certain times of their lives due to physiological, psychological, cultural or emotional factors.

Levels of adrenalin fall as soon as the stress subsides, but cortisol remains in the body much longer. This hormone sends a message to the brain to refuel, believing the body has used up large amounts of energy. As a consequence, you will eat more food than is actually necessary and put on weight. The deep fat cells in the belly are especially good at attracting cortisol, which causes them to release fat into the bloodstream and the excess to be stored as a layer of fat below the abdominal muscle. At the same time, the foods you often crave when you are stressed – biscuits, chocolate, cakes – raise blood sugar and therefore levels of insulin. High levels of sugar and insulin encourage your body to store fat and lead to insulin resistance.

Ageing and menopause

From around the age of 30, muscle mass gradually decreases each year and, as muscle is metabolically very active, causes a decline in the body's overall metabolic rate. There is also a decline in the growth hormone as you age, which is thought to contribute to weight gain around the middle. Most women find that their weight starts to increase particularly around the perimenopause, the years leading up to the menopause. This is because fat helps in the production of oestrogen, which reduces during menopause. The body will attempt to keep oestrogen levels high by holding on to the fat.

Exercise and metabolism

Your metabolism slows down as you age and you need to boost it through exercise. Building muscles through strength training is also very important, as muscles are metabolically active and continue to burn calories even at rest. Between the ages of 40 and 50 you will lose around 0.5 kg (1 lb) of muscle per year, and women lose muscle mass faster than men. Physical activity also helps to control the production of stress hormones (see above).

Body fat percentage

Fat is less metabolically active than muscle, meaning it requires fewer calories to sustain it. This is why body fat percentage is so important for weight control: the higher your percentage of fat (and the smaller your percentage of muscle), the fewer calories you need to maintain your weight and therefore the easier it is to gain weight.

Sleep

Lack of sleep can also adversely affect appetite as levels of leptin drop and ghrelin rise. Serotonin is another hormone affected by sleep and stress, and is also a contributing factor in controlling your appetite.

Serotonin produces the 'feel good' factor. When levels of this hormone are low, depression and apathy are likely to set in alongside weight gain – the lower your serotonin, the more you eat. Low serotonin levels can lead to food cravings (particularly for refined carbohydrates), low energy levels and compulsive eating. Women naturally have less serotonin in their brains than men.

Pollutants

Every day your body is subjected to environmental pollutants. Found in the atmosphere you breathe, in food packaging, or sprayed on to and added to your food, these agrichemical residues and food additives are stored within your fat cells, disrupting your body's natural hormonal balance.

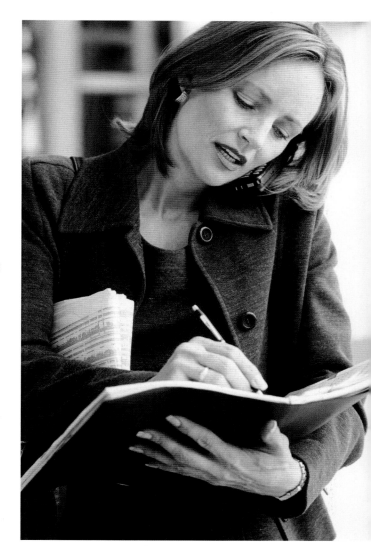

UNDERSTANDING DIET BASICS

To diet successfully you need to know the basic nutritional requirements of your body: a balance of carbohydrates, protein, healthy fats, fibre, minerals and vitamins, consumed in moderation. It is also helpful to understand the importance of keeping blood sugar levels steady and controlling portion size, as well as the counter-productive effects of calorie counting. The Waistline Diet Plan takes all these factors into consideration, offering nourishing menus that keep you feeling full even as you lose weight.

Carbohydrates

Carbohydrates give you energy to breathe, grow, move, function and repair. There are two types of carbohydrate: simple and complex. Simple carbohydrates provide sugar, some in a natural form as found in fruit and vegetables, others in refined form in foods such as cakes, biscuits and fruit squashes. Complex carbohydrates are starch based and are found in foods such as bread, cereals, pasta, rice, millet and pulses. Complex carbohydrates are healthier than simple carbohydrates.

Protein

Protein is required for growth and strength, as well as for muscle regeneration and hormone production. Protein is found in meat, poultry, eggs and fish, as well as in the vegetarian alternatives of tofu, nuts, seeds and pulses. It is also found in bread, rice and pasta.

Fibre

Fibre is necessary for the disposal of waste from the body. Particularly good sources are wholegrain bread and cereals, brown rice, vegetables, fruit, nuts and pulses.

Vitamins and minerals

Vitamins and minerals are vital for your body's everyday functioning. A balanced diet that includes wholegrains, fruit and vegetables, and fish, meat or pulses should provide you with your daily requirements. Choosing organic fruit and vegetables will help you to avoid the risk of residual pesticides. At certain times, such as during the menopause, you may consider taking a vitamin and mineral supplement.

Fats

Weight-for-weight, fat provides twice as many calories as carbohydrates or protein. If you eat too much, it is stored as adipose tissue – fat around the middle. Polyunsaturated and monounsaturated fats have the same calorie content as saturated fats, but are better for your health.

- **Saturated fat** This sort of fat is largely responsible for obesity, raised levels of 'bad' LDL cholesterol, hardening of the arteries, heart disease, some cancers and strokes. It also stimulates over-production of oestrogen, which can result in premenstrual and hormonal problems. Cutting down will help you to lose weight and keep you healthier. Saturated fat should be eaten only in moderation in foods such as eggs, grilled bacon, lamb, beef and hard cheese.
- **Polyunsaturated fat** This fat supplies the body with vitamins A, D and E, helps your hormones to stay in balance, supports your immune system, stimulates the metabolism, improves mood and brain function and keeps cell membranes healthy and joints supple. It is found in liquid fats and oils, including vegetable oil, corn oil and sunflower oil (palm oil should be avoided). It contains the essential fatty acids (EFAs) omega-3 and omega-6. You need to consume a variety of EFAs.

- **Omega-6** (linoleic fatty acid) is found mainly in oils including hemp, walnut, soya and wheatgerm, and in seeds such as pumpkin and sesame.
- **Omega-3** (alpha linoleic fatty acid) is found in oily fish like salmon, herring, tuna, sardines, kippers and mackerel, oils such as rapeseed, soya and linseed (an especially good source), nuts and seeds, green leafy vegetables, wholegrains and spirulina (seaweed).
- **Monounsaturated fat**, also known as omega-9, is also found in liquid form, but can solidify when cooled. It offers the benefits of polyunsaturated fat and also lowers levels of 'bad' LDL cholesterol and raises levels of 'good' high-density lipoprotein (HDL) cholesterol. It is linked to lower rates of heart disease and some cancers. Olive oil is the best source of this fat, along with rapeseed and sesame seed oils, avocados and olives themselves.
- **Trans fats** are 'good' vegetable fats that have been altered by food processing to improve their shelf life, texture and flavour. Often labelled as hydrogenated fats or hydrogenated vegetable oil, they are found in cakes, biscuits, pies, pastries, margarines and takeaways. They are as harmful as saturated fats to health, so try to cut them out altogether.

FAT-REDUCTION STRATEGIES

No more than 30 per cent of your total daily calorie intake should come from fat sources. 1 g of fat provides 9 calories, so, in a diet of 1500 calories per day, your total fat intake should not exceed 50 g (2 oz), with no more than 10 per cent of this being saturated fat. Here are some tips for reducing fat intake:

- Replace full-fat milk with skimmed, semi-skimmed or soya milk.
- Use butter and spreads sparingly.
- If using mayonnaise on bread, don't add butter or another spread as well.
- Steam, grill or poach foods, rather than frying.
- Avoid takeaway foods.
- Cut off the surplus fat from meat.
- Remove the skin from poultry.
- Limit your consumption of hard and full-fat cheeses.

COUNTING CALORIES

We all know that to lose weight you need to eat fewer calories, and use up the calories you do eat (this is especially true as you get older and your metabolism slows down). To lose weight sensibly, women should consume around 1,500 calories per day and men 2,000 calories per day. The average to maintain weight is 2,000 calories per day for women and 2,500 for men. However, all too often diets that offer a quick weight loss by cutting calories drastically can be difficult to maintain and leave you feeling deprived, depressed and miserable.

Low-calorie foods often adversely affect your blood sugar levels. For example, a breakfast of coffee, skimmed milk and low-calorie cereal may be a slimming meal, but the foods themselves are simple carbohydrates, lacking in fibre and protein. Once eaten they will be broken down quickly, blood sugar will rise dramatically and then fall just as quickly, leaving you feeling hungry around mid-morning and likely to snack. Many processed 'diet' foods are also full of chemicals and preservatives. The menus in the Waistline Diet Plan are built around wholesome, fresh foods that are high in nutritional value and won't leave you feeling empty.

GLYCAEMIC INDEX

When you eat, the food is converted into glucose that your body uses for energy. It is the hormone insulin that controls levels of glucose, storing it when there is too much in the body and releasing it when there is too little. If glucose levels are too high, high levels of insulin (see page 12) are released and the excess glucose is quickly

PORTION CONTROL

It's easy to eat too much. If you do, the chances are you won't feel any fuller, but you will pile on the extra weight. A good guide is that your plate should consist of one-half vegetables, one-quarter protein and one-quarter carbohydrates. A single helping should consist of:

Cooked rice or pasta	Fist-size portion
Meat, fish or poultry	Palm-size portion
Nuts	Tightly cupped hand-size portion
Raw vegetables	125 g (4 oz)
Cooked vegetables	60–70 g (2–2½ oz)
Fruit	Single fruit such as banana, apple, orange or pear; a cupped handful of strawberries, cherries or grapes; 3 plums; 4 apricots

stored away as fat. If you eat foods that raise glucose levels too high, you will produce too much insulin, increase your fat stores and gain weight. You may also develop insulin resistance. Conversely, if you choose foods that are slow to raise glucose levels this will help to keep insulin production under control.

The glycaemic index (GI) tells you how quickly a food raises blood sugar levels. Foods that are converted more slowly into glucose have a low GI value, while those causing a rapid and massive rise in blood sugar have a high GI value. Foods that break down quickly in the body – such as white bread, white rice and sugary treats – have the highest GI, while foods that take longer to be digested – such as new potatoes, wholewheat pasta and granary bread – have a lower GI.

The theory behind diets based on the glycaemic index is that foods with a low GI value release sugar slowly into the blood, providing you with a steady supply of energy that keeps you feeling satisfied for longer, so that you're less likely to snack. In contrast, foods with a high GI value cause a rapid but short-lived rise in blood sugar levels. This leaves you lacking in energy and feeling hungry again within a short time, so that you end up reaching for another carbohydrate 'fix'. It is these highs and lows that result in hunger and excess weight gain.

FOODS TO FIGHT MIDDLE-AGE SPREAD

Some foods are especially beneficial in combating middle-age weight gain and promoting good health and wellbeing. The menus in the Waistline Diet Plan are built around foods that will help to control the hormones, such as cortisol and insulin, that are associated with weight gain. The ingredients used in the meals will also help to reduce the effects of stress and pollution, and they will boost your metabolism, increasing the rate at which you burn off calories.

REGULATING HORMONES

The body's endocrine system is responsible for releasing chemical messengers – better known as hormones – into the bloodstream. Unfortunately, your hormones can be disrupted easily. Gaining weight, particularly around your middle, is linked to stress-related disruption of cortisol, which is secreted from the adrenal glands. Another factor in weight gain is overproduction of insulin, caused by an excess of blood sugar. (See pages 12–13 for more on the role of hormones.) Synthetic chemicals found in agrichemicals, food additives and preservatives, plastic packaging and so on also disrupt the body's endocrine system, by mimicking natural hormones.

Foods to balance hormones

A healthy diet helps to balance the endocrine system. Broccoli, for example, is a great source of chromium, a trace mineral that helps the pancreas to function properly and therefore increases insulin efficiency, which in turn helps to regulate blood sugar levels. Other foods you should include in your diet are:

- **Complex carbohydrates** Wholegrains, bread, rice, pulses, leafy green vegetables.
- **Vitamin B3** Yeast extract, wheat bran, turkey, chicken, fish, wholegrains, mushrooms, milk products.
- **Vitamin B6** Meat and dairy products, bananas, broccoli, red kidney beans, cauliflower, cabbage, watercress.
- **Zinc** Beef, lamb, calf's liver, turkey, sardines, crab, oyster, Brazil nuts, eggs, pumpkin seeds, yeast.
- **Protein** Chicken, meat, fish, eggs, milk, tofu, soya, quinoa.
- **Essential fatty acids (EFAs)** Oily fish, olive oil, nuts and seeds.

Foods to control insulin production

When you eat carbohydrates, your body responds by producing the hormone insulin. Good carbohydrates (see pages 14–16) are the key to keeping insulin production under control and the weight off. They are found in brown and basmati rice, oats, rye, millet, pulses, cherries, apples, pears, grapefruit, oranges, plums, dried apricots, green vegetables (leafy green ones, as well as courgettes, marrow, green peppers, cucumber, artichokes, celery), onions, garlic and tomatoes.

Foods to control stress hormones

Stress affects your adrenal glands by changing the behaviour of adrenal hormones (see pages 12–13). These hormones are responsible for many symptoms of stress, such as high blood pressure, digestive upset, muscle tension and, of course, fat around the middle. If the stress continues for a period of time, the adrenal glands can become exhausted. Foods high in nutrients that support adrenal gland function include:

- **Celery** Helps you to sleep if eaten at night; also helps to lower blood pressure.
- **Brown rice** Complex carbohydrate that helps to release serotonin, the feel-good, calming chemical that lifts mood and boosts energy.
- **Cabbage** Full of the antioxidant vitamins A, C and E, beta-carotene and the mineral selenium. Also releases serotonin for mood-boosting effects.
- **Sunflower seeds** Rich in vitamin B, zinc and potassium, all of which are heavily depleted by stress.
- **Berries** Rich in manganese and vitamin C to boost the immune system.

- **Avocados** Packed with beneficial polyunsaturated fats and minerals that stimulate the growth hormone and boost the metabolism.
- **Asparagus** Rich in the enzymes that help to regulate mood swings.
- **Sesame seeds** Source of zinc and useful in the metabolism of fatty acids and serotonin.

FIGHTING POLLUTION

Anitoxidants include vitamins A, C and E, selenium, carotenoids and phytochemicals. These substances protect your body against the damaging effects of an excess of 'free radicals', sources of which include pollution, sunlight, tobacco fumes, radiation, stress and illness. Excess free radicals cause cell damage and this is thought to lead to an increased risk of cancer, heart disease and arthritis. Antioxidants in your diet help to neutralize the free radicals in your body and halt their damaging effects.

- **Fruit and vegetables** Eat a wide variety – including sweet potatoes, carrots, spinach and mangoes – to provide you with plenty of antioxidants.
- **Green tea** This helps to protect your organs and flushes out toxins and pollutants.
- **Milk thistle** Use a supplement to protect your liver from toxins.

THE ROLE OF METABOLISM

Your metabolism is the rate at which your body burns calories in order to keep itself alive and it is always working, even when you are sleeping. Encouraging your metabolism to work more effectively is therefore a key factor in losing weight.

After the age of 30, your metabolic rate begins to drop by around 1 per cent each year, and as a result older dieters often complain that they cannot lose weight. But your metabolism can be boosted – you just need to know how and when.

How to boost metabolism

Your metabolism has 3 different aspects: the basal or resting metabolism; the activity metabolism; and the thermic or digestive metabolism. To boost your metabolism efficiently, you need to raise all 3 metabolic rates. To do this you need to:

- Eat first thing in the morning to kick-start your metabolism, and eat regularly throughout the day to prevent peaks and troughs in insulin production and carbohydrate metabolism (see pages 12–13).
- Exercise to build muscle and stimulate the growth hormone, as this helps to raise your basal metabolism. Any exercise also boosts your activity metabolism.
- Eat foods that contain protein, fibre, calcium and spices to boost your thermic and basal metabolisms.

Foods to boost metabolism

Certain foods take more energy to digest them, so it is worth including these in your diet to help to speed up your metabolism:

- **Complex carbohydrates** release energy slowly and boost your metabolism by keeping insulin levels low after you eat.
- **Calcium** Milk is one of the best foods for providing calcium, which boosts your basal metabolism. Other dairy products and leafy green vegetables are also good sources.
- **Protein** Protein is harder to digest than other food groups, so more energy is used by the body to break it down and therefore more calories are consumed.
- **Omega-3 oils** These alter the levels of leptin in the body, a hormone directly related to metabolism and responsible for whether you burn or store fat (see page 12). Low levels of leptin mean you burn more fat, and omega-3 reduces leptin levels. If you really don't like fish, or are vegetarian, then you can take an essential fatty acid supplement.
- **Fibre** Foods high in fibre boost your metabolism, as they take longer to digest.
- **Capsaicin** Found in peppers, this really raises your metabolism as it speeds up your heart rate. Peppers make a great snack option and the effect of capsaicin persists for several hours after you have finished

eating. It is also found in chilli spices, which you can add to your food.

- **Chromium** This trace mineral works with insulin to metabolize fats and carbohydrates, and a deficiency can cause blood sugar to soar and fat/carbohydrate metabolism to drop radically. Adding a chromium supplement to your diet will help to stabilize your blood sugar levels.
- **Water** Dehydration slows your thermic metabolism – you need water in your stomach in order to digest food. Aim to drink 8 glasses or 2 litres (4 pints) of fluid per day. Drinking enough water may be hard, but fruit juice can be a source as well as herbal tea.
- **Green tea** This type of tea contains a phytochemical known as ECGC, which researchers believe can boost your basal metabolism.

PLANNING AND MOTIVATION

You may have bought this book because you have a special party or holiday coming up and you want to look great in that new dress or bikini. Or maybe your health is suffering and you realize it is time to take stock, or perhaps you feel down and depressed. Whatever your reasons for starting the Waistline Plan, you will find that following it brings a whole range of different benefits, including increased energy, a positive frame of mind and a guilt-free attitude to food – not to mention a new waistline!

MAKE THAT COMMITMENT

For the initial 6 weeks of the Waistline Plan, make a commitment to your body and your health and fitness. Look at the Waistline Plan as being the most important thing in your life for the next 6 weeks: if you are totally committed to it, you will be surprised at how easily others accept your plans.

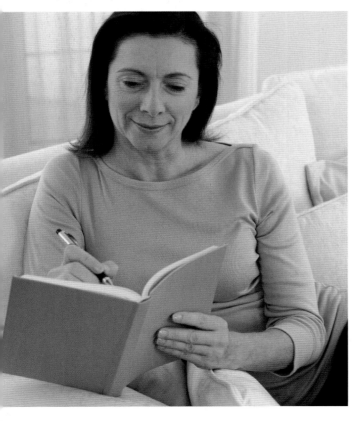

Set attainable goals, write them down and leave them in a place where you can see them every day, like on the door of the refrigerator or next to the phone. It's a good idea to set both short- and long-term goals, so you can cross off the short-term ones as you achieve them. Simple goals, such as not eating chocolate for 4 days or exercising for 10 minutes every day, may not sound much to others, but they will have a positive effect and make you realize just what you can achieve.

GOOD PLANNING

Planning ahead at every stage is the key to motivation and will help you to overcome any obstacles. Set a day to start, but preferably not a Monday – halfway through the week is much better psychologically. Avoid booking in any heavy social engagements or holidays during the first few weeks, which would impose extra pressure on you, and don't accept offers that may sabotage your efforts, such as an outing to a restaurant.

Empty your refrigerator and kitchen cupboards of all the food that is simply no good for you. Out go all processed foods such as white bread, biscuits, cakes, crisps, sweets, crackers, white pasta, white rice and sauces, along with ready meals and anything that isn't fresh and fruity. Stock up on the items listed on the shopping list (see page 26) before you start the plan, buying fresh fruit, vegetables, meat and fish as required during the course of the plan.

If you intend to swap days and meals around, plan this out on a weekly schedule and pin it up where you can see it easily. Include your snacks in the list and have them readily to hand or if necessary make them up, especially if you will be out and about for the day.

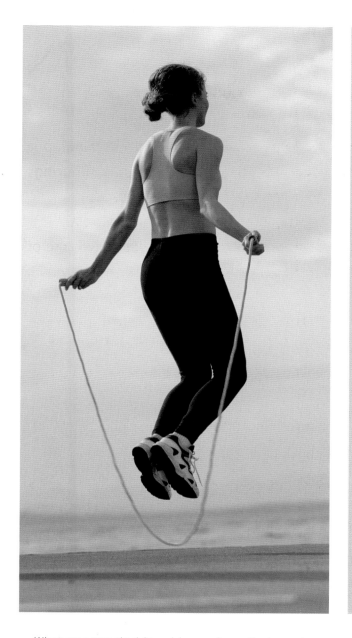

Like any new regime, there may be times when you find the Waistline Plan challenging. Here are some tips for keeping going:

• Make a list of all the reasons you are doing the Waistline Plan and put it somewhere where you will see it every day.

• Build in some rewards: celebrate the completion of the first week with a massage, manicure or trip to the cinema.

• Boost your metabolism by climbing stairs, skipping and walking that extra mile. The fitter you become, the easier it will be to follow the Waistline Plan.

• Exercising with a friend or partner will increase your commitment and make you work harder.

• Buy some attractive new workout wear to make exercise even more enjoyable.

• Think positively about exercise. If you experience a negative thought, push it away with a positive affirmation such as 'This will reduce my waistline'.

• Vary your workouts to keep them fresh.

• Chart your success, keeping a record of what you have eaten, how many times you have exercised and how much weight you have lost. Measure your chest, waist, hips and each thigh before you begin the plan, every other week during the plan, and again when you have completed it.

Whenever you start to get low on ingredients, make another shopping list and stick to it. If necessary, try internet shopping so that you won't be tempted by other foods when you get into the store.

Plan your toning and aerobic workouts for the week, then write them down in a simple chart form and pin this up beside your menu plan. Make sure you specify the times when you intend to work out on the chart and on your calendar – make a promise to yourself that you won't miss any of them. The best time to exercise is in the morning, as this will boost your metabolism for the rest of the day. Remember: you can fit in that extra 10 minutes if you want to! It's a good idea to stick to the same times

each day to exercise. If you get into a regular routine it will be easier to maintain.

You can always set yourself some personal exercise targets, such as adding another 10-minute exercise session into each day for the last week. Plan how you will treat yourself if you meet your targets; this will encourage you and help you to recognize your success.

If you really can't find time to exercise, perhaps because of unusually heavy work commitments, then at least try to walk further that day. Park the car away from the office, walk to the shops or in the park at lunchtime. Walk briskly to maximize the benefits. There are always ways to exercise a little more!

THE WAISTLINE

| 1 | 2 | 3 | 4 | 5 | 6 | 7 | 8 | 9 | 10 | 11 | 12 | 13 |

DIET PLAN

14 15 16 17 18 19 20 21 22 23 24 25 26

HOW THE DIET PLAN WORKS

The Waistline Diet Plan is not, in fact, a restrictive 'diet', but a positive change in your eating habits. You don't have to count calories all the time – just eat sensibly from a range of menu options, following the guidelines about portion size and ingredients. Feeding and nourishing your body properly, combined with taking more exercise, will help to boost your metabolism, stabilize blood sugar levels and regulate hormones. This is the only successful way of losing that excess weight around your middle.

WHAT DOES THE PLAN OFFER?

The Waistline Diet Plan sets out the next 42 days for you. Decide when you want to start, plan ahead using the shopping list on page 26, then follow the daily menus. These will provide the nutritious and balanced diet you need to lose that excess weight around your middle.

For convenience, you can occasionally mix and match meals on different days. For example, you may want to replace dinner on day 3 with dinner on day 10, or lunch on day 7 with lunch on day 12 – but do not replace a lunch with an extra dinner, or vice versa.

Nourishing your body

When you embark on the Waistline Diet Plan, you should eat a breakfast, lunch and dinner option and the snacks from each day's menu. Note that the dessert course applies to both main course alternatives, unless two desserts have been specified (in that case go with the dessert option that accompanies your chosen main course). The menus provide the right quantities of carbohydrate, protein, fats, vitamins, minerals and fibre for your daily needs. They also contain the ingredients that fight the causes of middle-age spread (see pages 12–13). You will be eating foods that balance hormones, control insulin production, counteract the effects of stress and pollution and boost your metabolism.

Meal schedule

When following the Waistline Diet Plan, you will be eating little and often. This will help to stabilize your blood sugar levels and prevent cravings for carbohydrates and sweet things. Ideally, you should try to eat your dinner before

7.30 pm. This will allow your body time to digest your meal before going to bed, helping you to sleep better.

The Waistline Diet Plan includes two healthy snacks each day. If you get really hungry, choose another snack or a fruit smoothie (these are really filling) from the plan.

Fruit and vegetables

Suggestions are given in the menus for the types of fruit, vegetables, nuts and seeds you can eat as snacks or to accompany a meal. This is simply to give you ideas that you might not otherwise have considered, but you can always create your own list (see the good foods discussed on pages 14–19). If possible, buy organic, fresh foods because these are the healthiest – food that is covered in pesticides and herbicides and full of additives can upset your hormonal balance and immune system.

Do not eat more than 5 pieces of fruit a day. Fruit contains its own sugar and this can ultimately affect your blood sugar levels.

Making life easy

As well as buying in the healthy ingredients you'll be using, it really is a good idea to get rid of all the foods you won't be eating. Having biscuits, cakes and pastries loitering in your cupboards will make temptation much harder to resist.

If you are catering for a family, you need to prepare them too, so that they can help to support you. The Waistline Diet Plan is not just healthy, it's designed to fit into your lifestyle and it's suitable for all the family. There are lots of vegetarian options, so you should find that there's something to please everyone.

GETTING THE MOST FROM THE PLAN

- Start the day with a drink of hot water and lemon to stimulate your liver and clean out toxins from your body.

- Always eat breakfast to kick-start your metabolism for the day.
- Try to build exercise session(s) into your morning schedule, as this will raise your metabolic rate and helps to burn fat throughout the day.
- Avoid coffee and alcohol. Cut back on your tea intake, too – try herbal teas instead.
- Turn off the television, put down the newspaper and don't look at the computer screen when you eat. It is very important to register what you are eating.
- Plan ahead: make sure you have all the foods for your menu in your store cupboard and refrigerator.
- Do not weigh yourself daily: once a week is plenty. Remember always to weigh yourself at the same time of day.
- Treat yourself every now and then. If you have been sticking to the plan for several weeks, then allow yourself a treat – but in moderation.
- Never eat late at night – it's not good for your digestion and may interrupt your sleep.
- Get enough sleep – it helps you to burn fat.

STAY HYDRATED

Remember that you can often mistake dehydration for hunger. Drink 6–8 glasses (1.5–2 litres/3–4 pints) of water per day. Your body is 70 per cent fluid, a proportion of which is lost through sweat, urine and breathing each day, so you need to replace it by drinking at regular intervals. Drink more water before, during and after exercise as well.

SHOPPING LIST

Before you begin the Waistline Diet Plan it is important to prepare yourself properly. Each day is planned, so that you know what you'll be eating and when. If you have the right ingredients to hand, there is much less chance of you snacking on something unsuitable. Below is a list of the basic foods that you'll require to follow the Waistline Diet Plan. Buy them in advance and replace them as necessary. Fresh fruit, vegetables, meat and fish are best bought as needed during the plan and used within a few days.

CEREALS
- Cereal (crunchy oat, wholegrain breakfast)
- Muesli (sugar-free)
- Oats (jumbo, rolled)

GRAINS
- Bagels
- Bread (multigrain, rye, wholegrain)
- Bulgar wheat
- Couscous
- Malt loaf
- Millet
- Noodles (buckwheat, thread egg)
- Pasta (egg, wholemeal)
- Pearl barley
- Pittas (wholemeal)
- Quinoa
- Rice (brown, wild)
- Rice pancakes

PULSES
- Beans (butter, flageolet, kidney, pinto)
- Lentils (Puy, red)
- Peas (chickpeas, split yellow peas)
- Tofu

NUTS
- Almonds
- Brazil nuts
- Cashew nuts
- Hazelnuts
- Pine nuts
- Walnuts

SEEDS
- Flax
- Pumpkin
- Sesame
- Sunflower

DRIED FRUIT
- Apricots
- Dates
- Prunes
- Raisins
- Sultanas

DAIRY PRODUCTS
- Butter
- Cheese (Cheddar, cottage cheese, low-fat cream cheese, feta, low-fat goat's, mozzarella, Parmesan, ricotta)
- Crème fraîche, low-fat
- Eggs
- Fromage frais
- Yogurt (low-fat Greek, natural or fruit)

DRINKS
- Fruit juices (apple, apple and mango, grapefruit, orange, pineapple, pomegranate, tomato)
- Milk (semi-skimmed or skimmed)
- Soya milk
- Tea (green, herbal)
- Water (filtered, mineral)

COOKING ALCOHOL
- Calvados
- Vodka
- White wine

OILS
- Chilli-infused
- Groundnut
- Olive
- Rapeseed
- Sesame
- Sunflower

GENERAL STORES
- Almond extract
- Artichoke hearts, canned
- Berry fruits, frozen
- Capers
- Chocolate, dark
- Cream of tartar
- Flour (buckwheat, wholemeal)
- Honey (clear)
- Hummus
- Mayonnaise, low-calorie
- Mirin
- Miso
- Mustard
- Oatcakes
- Olive oil spread
- Olives
- Orange-blossom water
- Peas, frozen
- Peanut butter
- Plum sauce
- Rice cakes
- Soy sauce
- Stock (chicken, fish, vegetable)
- Sugar (caster, light brown, light cane)
- Sun-dried tomatoes
- Tabasco sauce
- Tahini
- Thai fish sauce
- Tomato purée
- Tomatoes, canned
- Tuna, canned
- Vegetable soup, canned
- Vinegar (balsamic, cider, rice wine, white wine)
- Wasabi
- Water chestnuts, canned

SPICES
- Allspice berries
- Black mustard seeds
- Black peppercorns
- Cardamom
- Cayenne pepper
- Chilli powder
- Cinnamon
- Cloves
- Coriander seeds
- Cumin seeds
- Fennel seeds
- Garam masala
- Ground coriander
- Ground cumin
- Ground mace
- Ground turmeric
- Lemon pepper
- Nutmeg
- Onion seeds
- Paprika
- Rock salt
- Saffron threads
- Star anise

FOODS TO AVOID

These foods are the real villains. They can lead to excess weight gain, bloating, cellulite, erratic blood sugar levels and cravings. When you stop eating these foods, for the first few days you may find you experience headaches and cravings, but persevere and you will soon feel more energized, vibrant, healthy and awake. Your skin will improve, too.

- White bread
- White pasta
- White rice
- Refined cereals
- Sugar
- Cakes
- Scones
- Pastries
- Croissants
- Biscuits
- Chocolate
- Sweets
- Ice cream
- Crisps
- Saturated fats – avoid fried or processed foods
- Trans fats – avoid foods labelled hydrogenated fats or oil
- Ready meals
- Artificial flavourings, preservatives and additives
- Tea
- Coffee
- Fizzy drinks
- Fruit squash
- Alcohol

DIET MAINTENANCE PLAN

When you have finished the 6 weeks of diet and exercise, you will not only be seeing your results but feeling them too! Don't worry if you still have a little way to go before your stomach is as toned as you would like it to be: you have already done really well in getting this far, and by staying within the Waistline Diet Plan guidelines you will reach your goal. You have put in a lot of effort and commitment so far; keep up the good work with the Diet Maintenance Plan.

A PLAN FOR LIFE

If your weight is now where you want it to be, all you have to do is maintain it. If it's not quite there yet, then simply repeat the Waistline Diet Plan again.

You can use the Waistline Diet Plan as the basis for maintaining your ideal weight rather than losing any more. Start by simply adding in a few extras: for example, increase your portion of porridge for breakfast, introduce semi-skimmed rather than skimmed milk or have an extra smoothie during the day. You can also substitute in some favourite healthy recipes of your own.

Take care not to overdo the extras, particularly in the early days. You will find that if you re-introduce alcohol, for example, this will quickly increase your calorie intake and you may put on weight.

Maintaining the new you means changes for life. It really won't be as hard as you imagine, so believe in yourself and enjoy the journey.

KEEPING GOING

It can be all too easy to slip back into old habits, so keep reminding yourself that healthy eating is part of your new regime. Fortunately, there are lots of ways of maintaining your new look and healthy lifestyle.

- Keep a food diary and record everything you eat and drink. Don't cheat: the only person who stands to lose is you.
- Eat regular small, healthy meals and snacks every day.
- Eat breakfast, every day: you will be healthier and less likely to consume extra calories during the day.
- Continue to eat a healthy, balanced diet.
- Only eat refined foods occasionally.
- Drink plenty of water daily.
- Prepare your lunch in advance.
- Write a shopping list and stick to it.
- Get outside in the fresh air every day, even if it is just for a short walk.
- Make some time to exercise every day – as little as 10 minutes will still be beneficial.
- Reduce stress levels – the hormone cortisol needs to be kept in check (see page 12).
- Learn to breathe properly: it helps to reduce stress, lowers blood pressure and encourages weight loss.

Days 1 and 22

BREAKFAST

150 ml (¼ pint) glass of apple juice

Bowl of porridge
Make with 75 g (3 oz) rolled oats and 200 ml (7 fl oz) skimmed or soya milk, using 2 chopped, dried apricots or prunes to sweeten.

OR

150 ml (¼ pint) glass of pineapple juice

Large bowl of exotic fruit and 1 toasted bagel
Use fresh mango, pineapple and papaya, with a dash of orange juice and a sprinkling of sunflower seeds. Spread the bagel with 1 tablespoon low-fat cream cheese.

MID-MORNING SNACK

Handful of white grapes or an apple

LUNCH

2 hard-boiled eggs and salad
Season the eggs with paprika and use mixed salad leaves (rocket, baby spinach, radicchio) topped with 6 cherry tomatoes and dressed with 1 teaspoon olive oil mixed with lemon juice.

OR

Vegetable kebabs
Make up 2 skewers per person with seasoned tofu, mushrooms, peppers, courgette and onion, with a drizzle of olive oil. Grill for 5–10 minutes.

Strawberries or a pear

MID-AFTERNOON SNACK

2 oatcakes, topped with 1 teaspoon hummus

TIP OF THE DAY

From the day you begin the Waistline Diet Plan, keep a diary of how you feel. You may be surprised at how much healthier and more alert you are, and how your tastes for different foods change over the weeks.

DINNER

Seared tuna with lemony salsa
(see recipe)

OR

6–8 vegetarian nuggets per person with Vietnamese salad

Mix a salad of sliced carrots, spring onions and Chinese leaves, bean sprouts and chopped mint. Toss with a dressing of ½ tablespoon each sunflower oil, rice vinegar and light soy sauce and ½ teaspoon Thai fish sauce per person.

Berries with yogurt

For each person, spoon 2–3 tablespoons low-fat natural yogurt over a handful of strawberries, blueberries, blackberries and raspberries.

Seared Tuna with Lemony Salsa

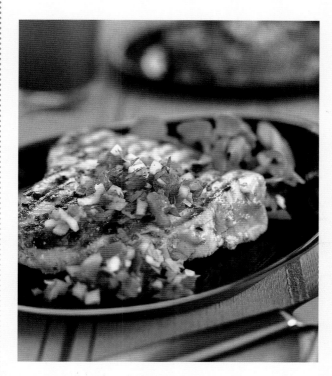

Preparation time:
30 minutes, plus marinating
Cooking time: 5 minutes
Serves 4

4 tuna steaks, about 400 g (13 oz) in total, cut about 1.5 cm (¾ in) thick
3 garlic cloves, finely chopped
1 teaspoon fennel seeds, finely ground
2 small dried red chillies, crumbled
1 tablespoon olive oil
4 tablespoons lemon juice

Salsa
250 g (8 oz) beef tomatoes, skinned, deseeded and finely chopped
1 small red onion, finely chopped
1 garlic clove, crushed
½ green chilli, deseeded and chopped
2 tablespoons lemon juice
grated rind from 1 unwaxed lemon
25 g (1 oz) coriander leaves, chopped
pinch of caster sugar

To garnish
handful of watercress leaves
grated rind from 1 unwaxed lemon

1 Place the tuna steaks on a chopping board and rub half the garlic into one side of the steaks, followed by half the ground fennel seeds and one of the chillies. Turn the steaks over and repeat the process on the other side with the remaining garlic, fennel and chilli.

2 Place the fish in a shallow container and pour over the olive oil and lemon juice. Cover and leave to marinate for 1 hour.

3 Meanwhile, make the salsa. Combine all the ingredients together in a bowl and then put it to one side to let the flavours develop.

4 Preheat a griddle or barbecue grill to very hot and sear the tuna for 1–2 minutes on each side. The tuna should be pink in the middle when it is served. If you prefer it cooked through, cook for an additional 2 minutes on each side.

5 Serve the tuna hot with the salsa, garnished with watercress leaves and the lemon rind. Accompany the tuna with mixed salad leaves (lettuce, endive, watercress).

NUTRITION

- Carbohydrate 5 g
- Fat 8 g
- Protein 25 g
- Energy 190 kcal (799 kJ)

Days 2 and 23

BREAKFAST

Mango and banana smoothie
Blend the flesh of 1 mango and 1 banana with 150 ml (¼ pint) skimmed milk, and add crushed ice.

OR

150 ml (¼ pint) glass of orange juice

Yogurt with muesli
Spoon 2 heaped tablespoons sugar-free muesli into 150 g (5 oz) low-fat fruit yogurt.

MID-MORNING SNACK

6 dried apricots or 3 fresh dates

LUNCH

Bean curry
Serves 2

Heat 2 teaspoons sunflower oil, add 1 teaspoon cumin seeds and let them pop for a few seconds. Stir in 1 tablespoon tomato purée, 1 teaspoon each ground spices (turmeric, coriander and cumin) and 2 teaspoons garam masala. Blend over a low heat. Mix in a 400 g (13 oz) can kidney beans, 2 sliced spring onions and 2 tablespoons chopped coriander leaves. Season with pepper and serve with brown rice.

OR

Tortillas
Serves 1

Make a salsa by combining 25 g (1 oz) ricotta cheese, ½ red onion, 1 tomato, ¼ green chilli and 1 tablespoon coriander, all finely chopped. Brush 2 flour tortillas with a little olive oil, then cook very briefly on each side on a griddle. Fill each tortilla with the salsa and serve with mixed salad leaves.

MID-AFTERNOON SNACK

2 rice cakes spread thinly with peanut butter

TIP OF THE DAY

Pulses such as kidney beans and split red lentils are high in soluble fibre, which helps to control glucose levels and regulate your appetite. They are also thought to lower blood cholesterol. Another reason to include a daily serving of these foods is that they contain phytoestrogens, which balance falling levels of oestrogen – common around the time of the menopause and a major cause of weight gain.

DINNER

**Jamaican chicken with
sweet potato wedges**
(see recipe)

OR

Red lentil dhal
Serves 4

Soak 225 g (7½ oz) red
lentils in warm water. Fry
1 onion, 2 cloves garlic, 1 cm
(½ in) fresh root ginger and
2 chillies, all chopped, for 3–
5 minutes. Stir in 4 chopped
tomatoes and soften. Add ½
teaspoon ground turmeric
and 1½ teaspoons garam
masala. Cover and simmer
for 5 minutes. Add the
drained lentils with 450 ml
(³⁄₄ pint) hot water and cook
for 15–20 minutes. Add salt,
4 tablespoons lemon juice
and chopped coriander.
Serve with brown rice.

Honeyed figs
Serves 4

Halve 8 fresh figs, drizzle
with honey and grill for
2–3 minutes. Garnish with
chopped flat-leaf parsley
and serve with raspberries
and 1 slice of low-fat goat's
cheese per person.

Jamaican Chicken with Sweet Potato Wedges

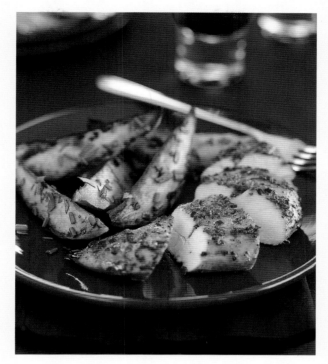

Preparation time:
20 minutes
Cooking time:
35–40 minutes
Serves 4

**4 skinless chicken breast
fillets, about 500 g (1 lb)
in total**

Jerk seasoning
8–10 allspice berries, crushed
**2 spring onions, green part
only, sliced**
4 garlic cloves, crushed
**1 cm (½ in) fresh root ginger,
peeled and shredded**
pinch of grated nutmeg
**2 pinches of ground
cinnamon**
1 teaspoon thyme
**1–2 Scotch Bonnet chillies,
deseeded and finely
chopped**
2 tablespoons soy sauce
juice of 2 limes

Sweet potato wedges
**2 orange-fleshed sweet
potatoes, about 750 g
(1½ lb) in total, unpeeled**
1 tablespoon olive oil
**2 tablespoons chopped
parsley**
**2 tablespoons chopped
chives**

1 Make the jerk seasoning. Mix the allspice berries with the
spring onions and pound until well mixed. Add the garlic,
ginger, nutmeg, cinnamon, thyme and chillies. Stir in the
soy sauce and lime juice and mix well. If necessary, add a
little water to bind.

2 Score the chicken breasts on both sides and rub in the
seasoning. Bake the chicken in a preheated oven, 190°C
(375°F), Gas Mark 5, for 30–40 minutes until it is crusty
on the outside.

3 Meanwhile, put the sweet potatoes in cold water and
bring to the boil. Cook the potatoes for 8–10 minutes until
parboiled, drain and leave to cool. Remove the skins and
cut into wedges.

4 Heat the oil in a nonstick pan and fry the wedges for
about 10 minutes until they are coloured on both sides.
Sprinkle with the parsley and chives and serve with the
cooked chicken cut into thick slices and mixed salad leaves
(rocket, lettuce, endive).

NUTRITION

- Carbohydrate 40 g
- Fat 7 g
- Protein 31 g
- Energy 343 kcal (1452 kJ)

Days 3 and 24

BREAKFAST

150 ml (¼ pint) glass of vegetable juice

Bowl of porridge
Make with 75 g (3 oz) rolled oats and 200 ml (7 fl oz) skimmed or soya milk, using 1 grated apple to sweeten.

OR

½ grapefruit

Boiled egg and 1 slice of wholegrain toast spread thinly with olive oil spread

TIP OF THE DAY

Flax seeds are high in omega-3 oils. They also contain phytoestrogens, which may help combat menopausal hot flushes and offer protection against breast cancer.

MID-MORNING SNACK

Small handful of nuts and seeds
Choose from almonds, Brazil nuts, hazelnuts, cashew nuts, pumpkin seeds, sunflower seeds or flax seeds.

LUNCH

Watercress soup
Serves 4

Fry 1 chopped onion until soft, add 100 g (3½ oz) watercress, 600 ml (1 pint) vegetable stock, salt and pepper and 2 tablespoons brown rice. Simmer until the rice is tender, then purée. Stir in 300 ml (½ pint) semi-skimmed milk and 150 g (5 oz) low-fat natural yogurt and reheat gently. Serve with 1 slice wholegrain or rye bread.

OR

Omelette and salad
Make with 2 eggs and use mixed salad leaves (rocket, baby spinach, watercress), drizzled with lemon juice and olive oil.

MID-AFTERNOON SNACK

Apple, pear or nectarine

DINNER

Grilled sea bass
(see recipe)

OR

Mushroom stroganoff
Serves 4

Fry 1 sliced onion in 1½ tablespoons olive oil until lightly browned. Add 400 g (13 oz) sliced mushrooms and 2 finely chopped garlic cloves. Cook for 4 minutes, stir in 2 teaspoons paprika and cook for 1 minute. Add 6 tablespoons vodka. When bubbling, flame with a match. Once the flames subside, stir in 400 ml (14 fl oz) vegetable stock, a pinch each ground mace and ground cinnamon, and salt and pepper. Simmer for 4 minutes. Add 150 g (5 oz) sliced wild mushrooms and cook for 2 minutes. Stir in 2 tablespoons low-fat crème fraîche.

2 kiwifruit or 3 fresh apricots per person

Grilled Sea Bass

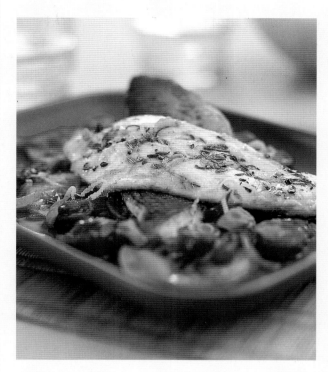

Preparation time:
15 minutes
Cooking time: 12–13 minutes
Serves 6

1 tablespoon olive oil
1 onion, finely chopped
300 g (10 oz) cherry
   tomatoes, halved
2 large pinches of saffron
   threads (optional)
150 ml (¼ pint) dry
   white wine
125 ml (4 fl oz) fish stock
grated rind of 1 lemon, the
   rest halved and thinly
   sliced
12 small sea bass fillets,
   about 100 g (3½ oz) each,
   rinsed in cold water
1 teaspoon fennel seeds
salt and pepper
basil or oregano leaves, to
   garnish (optional)

1 Heat the oil in a frying pan, add the onion and fry for 5 minutes until softened and lightly browned. Add the tomatoes, saffron (if using), wine and stock and stir in the lemon rind and a little salt and pepper. Bring to the boil and cook for 2 minutes.

2 Pour the mixture into the base of a foil-lined grill pan, add the lemon slices and set aside until ready to complete.

3 Arrange the fish fillets, skin side uppermost, on top of the tomatoes. Use a teaspoon to scoop some of the juices over the skin, then sprinkle with salt and pepper and the fennel seeds.

4 Cook under a preheated grill for 5–6 minutes until the skin is crispy and the fish flakes easily when pressed with a knife. Transfer to serving plates and sprinkle with basil or oregano leaves, if liked. Serve with steamed green vegetables (mangetout, courgette, broccoli).

NUTRITION

- Carbohydrate 4 g
- Fat 7 g
- Protein 39 g
- Energy 252 kcal (1057 kJ)

Days 4 and 25

BREAKFAST

150 ml (¼ pint) glass of apple juice

Bowl of muesli
Make with 75 g (3 oz) sugar-free muesli and 200 ml (7 fl oz) skimmed or soya milk, using 1 sliced banana to sweeten.

OR

150 ml (¼ pint) glass of apple or orange juice

Exotic fruit salad
Use melon, pineapple and mango and add 2 tablespoons low-fat natural yogurt.

MID-MORNING SNACK

Vegetable crudités with hummus
Use a handful of chopped, raw vegetables (carrots, cucumber, peppers, celery, cherry tomatoes) and 2 tablespoons hummus.

LUNCH

Ricotta, smoked salmon and artichoke wrap
(see recipe)

OR

Wholemeal pitta with turkey salad
Fill a pitta with tomatoes, lettuce, celery, cucumber, chopped spring onions and a slice of lean turkey breast, plus 1 tablespoon low-fat natural yogurt as dressing.

Pear or apple

MID-AFTERNOON SNACK

2 rice cakes spread thinly with tahini or cottage cheese

TIP OF THE DAY

Low serotonin levels are linked to depression and weight gain. Turkey, like bananas, is naturally high in serotonin.

DINNER

Peppered steak
Serves 2

Trim the fat from 2 thick-cut sirloin steaks (500 g/1 lb in total) and rub with crushed peppercorns and salt. Mix 200 g (7 oz) yogurt and 1 crushed garlic clove, add salt and pepper and toss with salad leaves and 1 sliced red onion. Fry the steaks in 1 tablespoon olive oil for 2 minutes. Turn over and cook for 2–5 minutes. Serve with the salad and roasted sweet potatoes.

OR

Sizzling tofu
Serves 2

Marinate 125 g (4 oz) tofu slices in sesame oil and soy sauce. Dry-fry some sesame seeds, place in a dish and pour the tofu marinade over them. Grill the tofu. Stir-fry 1 cm (½ in) fresh root ginger, 1 garlic clove, 1 shallot and 250 g (8 oz) pak choi, all chopped, in 1 tablespoon sunflower oil. Mix in ½ tablespoon each rice vinegar and soy sauce and the sesame seeds. Serve with the tofu.

1 melon slice per person

Ricotta, Smoked Salmon and Artichoke Wrap

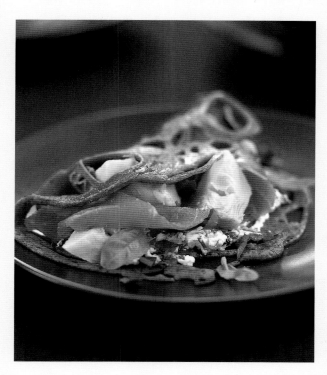

Preparation time: 20 minutes
Cooking time: 15 minutes
Serves 6

Batter
100 g (3½ oz) buckwheat flour
1 egg
250 ml (8 fl oz) semi-skimmed milk

Filling
125 g (4 oz) ricotta cheese
3 tablespoons chopped parsley or parsley and basil mixed, plus extra basil leaves to garnish
1 small garlic clove, crushed (optional)
grated rind of ½ lemon and juice of 1 lemon
2 tablespoons sunflower oil
250 g (8 oz) smoked salmon, sliced
400 g (13 oz) can artichoke hearts, drained and quartered
salt and pepper

1 Make the batter. Put the flour, egg, a little of the milk and some salt into a bowl and whisk until smooth. Gradually whisk in the remaining milk.

2 Make the filling. Mix the ricotta with the herbs, garlic (if using) and lemon rind and season gently.

3 Heat a little of the oil in a nonstick frying pan. When it is hot pour the excess into a small, heatproof bowl. Drizzle in 3 tablespoons of the batter to make lacy crêpes about 18 cm (7 in) in diameter, then cook until the underside is browned. Loosen with a palette knife, turn over and cook the other side in the same way. Lift the crêpe out on to a plate and keep warm. Make 5 more in the same way, adding more oil if needed.

4 Arrange each crêpe on a serving plate, divide the ricotta filling among them and top with strips of smoked salmon and artichoke quarters. Drizzle with lemon juice and sprinkle with pepper. Fold the crêpes over the filling and garnish with some extra chopped herbs.

NUTRITION

- Carbohydrate 19 g
- Fat 10 g
- Protein 19 g
- Energy 229 kcal (958 kJ)

Days 5 and 26

BREAKFAST

Strawberry and raspberry smoothie
Blend together ½ banana, 3 strawberries, 3 raspberries, 1 tablespoon low-fat natural yogurt and 150 ml (¼ pint) skimmed or soya milk.

OR

200 ml (7 fl oz) glass of apple juice

Boiled egg and 1 slice of wholegrain bread

MID-MORNING SNACK

Handful of white grapes or an apple

LUNCH

Miso broth
Serves 6

Simmer the following for 5 minutes: the white parts of 4 thinly sliced spring onions, 2 cm (¾ in) fresh root ginger, finely chopped, 1 sliced red chilli, 1.5 litres (2½ pints) fish or vegetable stock, 3 tablespoons chilled miso, 2 tablespoons mirin (Japanese cooking wine), 1 tablespoon soy sauce. Add the green parts of the spring onions, 100 g (3½ oz) pak choi, 2 tablespoons chopped coriander and 150 g (5 oz) cooked prawns. Cook until the pak choi has just wilted.

OR

Small baked potato with 125 g (4 oz) cottage cheese or tuna.

MID-AFTERNOON SNACK

Oven-baked crunchy chickpeas
Serves 2

Mix together 150 g (5 oz) can chickpeas, drained and rinsed, 1 teaspoon olive oil and a pinch each of rock salt, ground cumin, chilli powder and ground coriander. Place the mix on a baking sheet and bake in a preheated oven, 200°C (400°F), Gas Mark 6, for 10–15 minutes until golden. Allow to cool before serving.

TIP OF THE DAY

Keep your refrigerator stocked up. This will help you to avoid snacking on unhealthy foods.

DINNER

Spanish fish stew
(see recipe)

OR

Mediterranean peppers
Serves 4

Fill 4 halved peppers with 24 halved cherry tomatoes, 2 sliced garlic cloves, 40 g (1½ oz) capers and basil leaves. Drizzle with olive oil and season. Pour some water into the base of the dish, cover with foil and cook in a preheated oven, 180°C (350°F), Gas Mark 4, for 20 minutes. Remove the foil, reduce to 150°C (300°F), Gas Mark 2, and bake for 40 minutes. Garnish with basil and serve with salad leaves.

Grilled pineapple and plum sauce
Serves 4

Simmer 425 g (14 oz) diced plums, 3 star anise and a pinch each ground chilli and cinnamon with 6 tablespoons water until soft. Grill the pineapple slices until lightly browned. Serve with the plum sauce.

Spanish Fish Stew

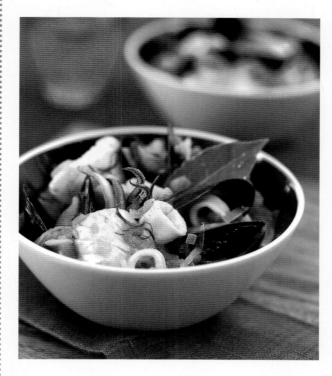

Preparation time:
30 minutes
Cooking time: 24 minutes
Serves 4

1 tablespoon olive oil
1 large onion, finely chopped
2 garlic cloves, finely chopped
½ teaspoon pimentón (smoked paprika)
500 g (1 lb) tomatoes, skinned and chopped
1 red pepper, cored, deseeded and diced
200 ml (7 fl oz) fish stock
150 ml (¼ pint) dry white wine
2 large pinches of saffron threads
4 small bay leaves
500 g (1 lb) fresh mussels, soaked in cold water
200 g (7 oz) cleaned calamari, rinsed in cold water
375 g (12 oz) cod loin, skinned
salt and pepper

1 Heat the oil in a large saucepan, add the onion and fry for 5 minutes until softened and just beginning to brown. Stir in the garlic and pimentón and cook for 1 minute.

2 Mix in the tomatoes, red pepper, fish stock, wine and saffron. Add the bay leaves, season to taste with salt and pepper and bring to the boil. Cover and simmer gently for 10 minutes. Set aside until needed.

3 Discard any mussels that are open or cracked. Scrub the shells with a nailbrush, remove any barnacles and pull off the hairy tuft-like beard. Return the mussels to a bowl of clean water. Separate the calamari tubes from the tentacles and slice the tubes. Cut the cod into cubes.

4 Reheat the tomato sauce if necessary, add the cod and the calamari slices and cook for 2 minutes. Add the mussels, cover and cook for 4 minutes. Add the calamari tentacles and cook for 2 minutes until cooked through and all the mussels have opened. Gently stir and spoon into bowls to serve.

NUTRITION

• Carbohydrate 11 g
• Fat 5 g
• Protein 32 g
• Energy 240 kcal (1009 kJ)

Days 6 and 27

BREAKFAST	MID-MORNING SNACK	LUNCH	MID-AFTERNOON SNACK

200 ml (7 fl oz) glass of pomegranate juice

Fresh fruit compote
Use kiwifruit, pineapple, papaya and mango. Top with 2 tablespoons low-fat natural yogurt and a sprinkling of sunflower seeds.

OR

150 ml (¼ pint) glass of chilled tomato juice

Savoury bagel
Spread the bagel with 1 tablespoon low-fat cream cheese and top with 25 g (1 oz) smoked salmon or wafer-thin honey-roast ham.

Nectarine or peach

Chicken salad Thai style (see recipe)

OR

Chickpea and olive salad
Serves 4

Stir together a drained 250 g (8 oz) can chickpeas, 50 g (2 oz) black olives, ½ chopped red onion, 150 g (5 oz) tomatoes and 3 tablespoons chopped flat-leaf parsley. Toss with a mixed dressing of 1 crushed garlic clove, 100 g (3½ oz) low-fat Greek yogurt and the juice of ½ lime, seasoned with pepper. Serve on a bed of watercress.

150 g (5 oz) low-fat natural yogurt with 1 teaspoon clear honey

1 slice of malt loaf

TIP OF THE DAY

Pomegranates are packed with vitamins C and E and folic acid. They have 3 times the antioxidant levels of tea or red wine — a glass of pomegranate juice per day can reduce the risk of developing cardiovascular disease.

DINNER

Grilled/poached salmon

Serve a 150 g (5 oz) salmon steak per person with steamed vegetables.

OR

Stir-fried noodles
Serves 4

Cook 225 g (7½ oz) thread egg noodles. Stir-fry 1 onion and 1 cm (½ in) fresh root ginger, both chopped, in 1 tablespoon groundnut oil for 2–3 minutes. Add 200 g (7 oz) chopped mushrooms and cook for 1–2 minutes. Add 125 g (4 oz) bean sprouts, 2 sliced red peppers, 1 tablespoon plum sauce, 2 tablespoons soy sauce and 6 sliced spring onions, and cook for a few minutes. Mix in the noodles.

Baked bananas

Slice 1 banana per person lengthways and wrap in foil with 1 tablespoon water, ½ tablespoon clear honey, ½ teaspoon lemon juice, 15 g (½ oz) raisins and a pinch of cinnamon. Bake in a preheated oven, 200°C (400°F), Gas Mark 6, for 10 minutes.

Chicken Salad Thai Style

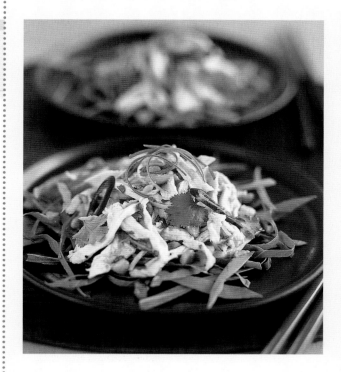

Preparation time:
10 minutes
Cooking time:
15–20 minutes
Serves 4

150 g (5 oz) cooked chicken breast, shredded
3 tablespoons coriander leaves
150 g (5 oz) pak choi, shredded

Dressing
1 tablespoon groundnut oil
1 tablespoon Thai fish sauce
juice of 1 lime
juice of 1 small orange
1 garlic clove, crushed
3 tablespoons roughly chopped basil leaves
pepper

To garnish
2 spring onions, green stems only, shredded lengthways
1 plump red chilli, deseeded and sliced diagonally

1 Make the dressing by shaking all the ingredients together in a screw-top jar.

2 Mix the chicken with the coriander leaves and then stir in the dressing.

3 Line a serving dish with the pak choi, spoon the dressed chicken on top and serve chilled, garnished with spring onion shreds and red chilli slices.

NUTRITION

• Carbohydrate 4 g
• Fat 7 g
• Protein 16 g
• Energy 144 kcal (604 kJ)

Days 7 and 28

BREAKFAST

Carrot and apple juice
Juice together 3 carrots, 2 apples and 2 sticks of celery.

Bowl of muesli
Make with 75 g (3 oz) sugar-free muesli and 200 ml (7 fl oz) skimmed or soya milk or 3 tablespoons low-fat natural yogurt, using 1 grated apple to sweeten.

OR

150 ml (¼ pint) glass of apple juice

2 scrambled eggs and 1 slice of wholegrain toast

MID-MORNING SNACK

6 dried apricots or 6 Brazil nuts

LUNCH

Bulgar wheat salad
Serves 2

Soak 125 g (4 oz) bulgar wheat for 30 minutes, then drain and squeeze dry. Add 4 sliced plums, 1 crushed garlic clove, 1 finely chopped red onion, a handful each chopped parsley and mint, 2 tablespoons olive oil and 4 tablespoons lemon juice. Add salt and pepper, and refrigerate for at least 30 minutes. Serve with 4 tablespoons low-fat yogurt, mixed with 1 crushed garlic clove, ½ teaspoon each cayenne pepper and tomato purée and some finely chopped chives.

OR

Wholemeal tuna pitta
Fill a pitta with a 185 g (6½ oz) can tuna, mixed salad leaves (radicchio, endive, rocket) and some chopped cherry tomatoes, red onion and parsley or coriander. Add a squeeze of lemon juice, 1 tablespoon low-fat natural yogurt and some chopped mint.

MID-AFTERNOON SNACK

2 pieces of fruit
Choose from apple, nectarine, satsuma, pear or a small handful of grapes.

TIP OF THE DAY

If you are eating out in a restaurant, go for the healthy option. Ask for the sauce to be served on the side and for there to be no dressing on salad and vegetables.

DINNER

Herby lamb
(see recipe)

OR

Lentil pilaf
Serves 4

Sauté 1 chopped garlic clove
and 1 chopped bunch spring
onions in 1 tablespoon olive
oil until soft. Add 125 g
(4 oz) lentils, 50 g (2 oz)
each brown rice and wild
rice and 600 ml (1 pint)
vegetable stock. Bring to the
boil, then turn down the
heat and simmer until nearly
all the stock has gone. Add
1 tablespoon each chopped
almonds and chopped
thyme. Serve with mixed
green leaves (baby spinach,
watercress, radicchio).

**1 sliced papaya
per person**

Herby Lamb

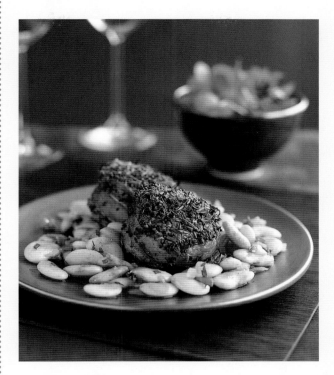

1 Mix together all the chopped herbs in a bowl. Spread
mustard on both sides of each noisette and dip the meat
into the herb mixture. Press the herbs firmly to the
mustard. Chill the lamb in the refrigerator until you are
ready to cook.

2 Make the tangy butter beans. Heat the oil in a frying pan
and fry the onion until it has softened. Add the remainder
of the ingredients to the frying pan and cook gently for
5 minutes.

3 Preheat the grill to hot and cook the lamb noisettes for
about 4 minutes each side. The lamb should be cooked but
still retain a slight pink colour.

4 Serve the lamb immediately, surrounded by the tangy
butter beans. Accompany with steamed green vegetables
(courgette, broccoli, cabbage, cauliflower).

Preparation time:
10 minutes
Cooking time:
15–20 minutes
Serves 4

**2 tablespoons finely
chopped mint**
**1 tablespoon finely chopped
thyme**
**1 tablespoon finely chopped
oregano**
**½ tablespoon finely chopped
rosemary**
**4 teaspoons wholegrain
mustard**
**4 lamb noisettes, about
125 g (4 oz) each**

Tangy butter beans
2 teaspoons sunflower oil
1 medium onion, chopped
**250 g (8 oz) cooked butter
beans or drained canned
beans**
1 tablespoon tomato purée
**50 ml (2 fl oz) pineapple
juice**
2 tablespoons lemon juice
**a few drops of Tabasco
sauce**
pepper

NUTRITION

- Carbohydrate 14 g
- Fat 14 g
- Protein 32 g
- Energy 305 kcal (1280 kJ)

Days 8 and 29

BREAKFAST

150 ml (¼ pint) glass of orange juice

Large fresh fruit salad
Use apple, pear, grapes and kiwifruit. Top with 2 tablespoons low-fat natural yogurt and a sprinkling of sunflower and flax seeds.

OR

150 ml (¼ pint) glass of apple juice

Bowl of wholegrain cereal
Make with 75 g (3 oz) wholegrain cereal and 150 ml (¼ pint) skimmed or soya milk.

MID-MORNING SNACK

Small handful of toasted nuts
Grill almonds, cashew nuts or walnuts, or a mixture of these, for 5–7 minutes.

LUNCH

Wholemeal pitta filled with 100 g (3½ oz) smoked trout and some watercress

OR

Vietnamese vegetable spring rolls
(see recipe)

150 g (5 oz) low-fat fruit yogurt per person

MID-AFTERNOON SNACK

2 oatcakes topped with 2 tablespoons low-fat cottage cheese

TIP OF THE DAY

Nuts are high in essential omega-3 and omega-6 oils. Full of vitamins and minerals, they help you to burn fat by speeding up your metabolism. The secret is not to eat too many of them!

DINNER

Grilled halibut
Serves 4

Brush 4 halibut steaks (625 g/1¼ lb total) with olive oil, season and grill until cooked. Stir-fry 1 teaspoon crushed fresh root ginger and ¼ teaspoon fennel seeds in 2 tablespoons olive oil for a few seconds. Add 500 g (1 lb) broccoli florets, 3 tablespoons soy sauce and pepper, and stir-fry until just cooked. Serve with the fish.

OR

Fruity couscous
Serves 4

Swell 200 g (7 oz) couscous in hot vegetable stock. Add 1 stir-fried chopped red onion and red pepper, 10 g (½ oz) each chopped parsley, basil and mint, the juice and rind of 1 lime, a pinch of ground cinnamon, 50 g (2 oz) chopped dried apricots and 25 g (1 oz) toasted flaked almonds. Serve with mixed salad leaves.

6 stewed prunes or 2 plums per person

Vietnamese vegetable spring rolls

Preparation time: 30 minutes
Cooking time: 5 minutes
Serves 4

200 g (7 oz) pak choi
2 tablespoons sunflower oil
100 g (3½ oz) sweet potato, cut into matchstick strips
100 g (3½ oz) carrot, cut into matchstick strips
½ bunch of spring onions, cut into matchstick strips
50 g (2 oz) bean sprouts, rinsed and drained
2 garlic cloves, finely chopped
2 cm (¾ in) piece of fresh root ginger, peeled and finely chopped
50 g (2 oz) or 8 rice pancakes
bunch of coriander

Sauce
4 ripe red plums, about 250 g (8 oz) in total
2 tablespoons water
1 tablespoon soy sauce
made-up wasabi (Japanese horseradish sauce), to taste
1 tablespoon caster sugar

1 Cut the leaves from the pak choi and slice the stems into thin matchstick strips. Heat 1 tablespoon of the oil in a wok or large frying pan, add the sweet potato and carrot and stir-fry for 2 minutes. Add the spring onions and pak choi stems and cook for 1 minute. Mix in the bean sprouts, garlic and ginger and cook for 1 minute. Transfer to a bowl.

2 Heat the remaining oil in the pan, add the pak choi leaves and cook for 2–3 minutes until just wilted.

3 Dip a rice pancake into a bowl of hot water and leave for 20–30 seconds until softened. Lift out and place on a tea towel. Top with a pak choi leaf, one-eighth of the vegetable mixture and 2 stems of coriander. Fold in the pancake edges and roll up tightly, repeating to make 8 pancakes in all. Cover with clingfilm and set aside. Serve within 1 hour.

4 Meanwhile, make the sauce. Stone and chop the plums. Place in a small saucepan with the water, cover and cook for 5 minutes until softened. Purée the plums with the soy sauce, then mix in the wasabi and sugar to taste.

5 Garnish the pancakes with the remaining sprigs of coriander and serve with small bowls of the sauce.

NUTRITION

- Carbohydrate 27 g
- Fat 6 g
- Protein 4 g
- Energy 176 kcal (734 kJ)

Days 9 and 30

BREAKFAST

Strawberry and banana smoothie
Blend together 1 banana, 6 strawberries and 200 ml (7 fl oz) chilled skimmed milk.

OR

150 ml (¼ pint) glass of orange juice

Bowl of porridge
Make with 75 g (3 oz) rolled oats and 200 ml (7 fl oz) skimmed or soya milk, adding 6 chopped strawberries to sweeten.

MID-MORNING SNACK

Vegetable crudités with hummus
Use a handful of chopped, raw vegetables (carrots, cucumber, peppers, celery, cherry tomatoes) and 2 tablespoons hummus.

LUNCH

Avocado salad and 1 slice of rye bread spread thinly with tahini
Slice ½ avocado on to a bed of mixed salad (watercress, baby spinach, radicchio, celery, cherry tomatoes, cucumber).

OR

Filled sandwich of wholegrain bread with olive oil spread
Fill with grilled chicken, mixed salad leaves (baby spinach, lamb's lettuce, radicchio) and some sliced tomato.

Apple or pear

MID-AFTERNOON SNACK

2 rice cakes spread with 2 tablespoons low-fat cream cheese

TIP OF THE DAY

Avocados are a good source of monosaturated fat. This sort of fat is known to maintain levels of good HDL cholesterol, which is associated with a lower risk of cardiovascular disease.

DINNER

Roast pepper and walnut pappardelle
(see recipe)

150 g (5 oz) low-fat natural yogurt

OR

Grilled chicken
Serve a grilled 150 g (5 oz) chicken breast per person with 125 g (4 oz) baked sweet potato and a tomato and red onion salad.

Strawberry whip
Blend together 1 banana, 5 strawberries and 1 tablespoon low-fat natural yogurt per person. Sprinkle with sunflower seeds.

Roast Pepper and Walnut Pappardelle

Preparation time:
10–15 minutes
Cooking time: 35 minutes
Serves 4

2 teaspoons olive oil
4 red peppers, cored, deseeded and sliced
3–4 large garlic cloves, thinly sliced
60 g (2½ oz) walnuts, chopped
300 g (10 oz) fresh egg pappardelle
25 g (1 oz) Parmesan cheese shavings
salt and pepper

1 Use ½ teaspoon of the olive oil to brush over the peppers. Put the peppers on a baking sheet and roast them in a preheated oven, 230°C (450°F), Gas Mark 8, for 20–25 minutes until they are soft and just beginning to blacken.

2 Reserve 4 slices of pepper to use as a garnish and cut the remaining peppers into large dice.

3 Heat the remaining olive oil in a large frying pan over a medium-low heat, add the sliced garlic but do not let it brown. Add the diced red pepper and stir in the walnuts. Keep warm.

4 Bring a large saucepan of lightly salted water to the boil. Add the pasta, return to the boil and cook for 3–4 minutes or until the pasta is *al dente*. Drain and transfer to a large, warm serving bowl.

5 Toss the pasta well with the garlic, pepper and walnut mixture. Sprinkle over the Parmesan shavings and garnish with the reserved pepper slices.

NUTRITION

- Carbohydrate 63 g
- Fat 16 g
- Protein 15 g
- Energy 435 kcal (1833 kJ)

Days 10 and 31

BREAKFAST

150 ml (¼ pint) glass of apple juice

2 large grilled tomatoes on 1 slice of wholegrain toast

OR

150 ml (¼ pint) glass of pineapple juice

Bagel spread with 25 g (1 oz) low-fat cream cheese, with 1 slice lean ham and 1 tomato.

MID-MORNING SNACK

2 pieces of fruit
Choose from apple, pear, orange, peach or nectarine.

LUNCH

Chicken and bean salad
Serves 2

Mix together 1 tablespoon lemon juice, 1 teaspoon olive oil and a pinch each of paprika and pepper to make the dressing. Mix together the salad ingredients: 50 g (2 oz) each cooked, sliced chicken breast, cooked kidney beans, cooked chickpeas; 25 g (1 oz) each finely sliced, cooked leeks, sliced red pepper, sliced mushrooms. Pour over the dressing and mix well. Serve on a bed of mixed salad leaves (baby spinach, rocket, lettuce).

OR

Tofu and bean salad
Make as above, substituting the chicken with grilled tofu.

MID-AFTERNOON SNACK

Small handful of pumpkin and sunflower seeds

TIP OF THE DAY

Tomatoes are a rich source of vitamins A and C. They also contain lycopene, an antioxidant that has been linked to a reduced risk of breast, pancreatic and ovarian cancers.

DINNER

Griddled artichokes and fennel
(see recipe)

Serve with a 150 g (5 oz) pan-fried salmon fillet or tuna steak and 50 g (2 oz) brown rice per person.

OR

Serve the artichokes with 125 g (4 oz) baked tofu and 50 g (2 oz) brown rice per person.

Baked pear with almond crumble
Serves 4

Mix 75 g (3 oz) wholemeal flour, 60 g (2½ oz) ground almonds and 75 g (3 oz) light brown sugar. Rub in 60 g (2½ oz) butter until it resembles fine breadcrumbs. Arrange 4 pears, unpeeled, cored and sliced lengthways, in 4 tall ovenproof ramekins and drizzle with the juice of 1 lime. Cover with the crumble and sprinkle over 2 tablespoons flaked almonds. Bake in a preheated oven, 220°C (425°F), Gas Mark 7, for 20 minutes. Serve warm, topped with crème fraîche, if liked.

Griddled Artichokes and Fennel

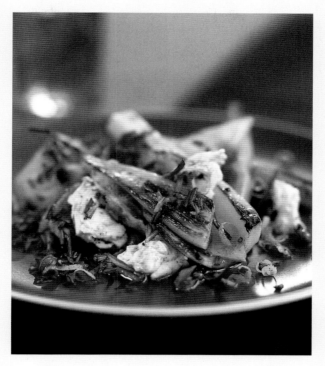

Preparation time:
15 minutes
Cooking time: 7–8 minutes
Serves 6

3 tablespoons olive oil
3 teaspoons finely chopped rosemary leaves
200 g (7 oz) fennel heads, stems separated and any large pieces halved
400 g (13 oz) can artichoke hearts, drained and halved
100 g (3½ oz) feta cheese, drained and crumbled
sprigs of rosemary, to garnish

Dressing
grated rind and juice of 1 lemon
2 teaspoons capers, drained
4 teaspoons balsamic vinegar
salt and pepper

1 Put the oil, chopped rosemary and a little salt and pepper in a plastic bag. Add the fennel and artichoke hearts and shake gently in the bag.

2 Heat a ridged frying pan, add the dressed vegetables and cook for 3–4 minutes until the undersides are browned. Turn them over and cook for 2 minutes. Crumble the cheese over the top and place the pan under a preheated grill for 2 more minutes until the cheese is hot but not melted.

3 Meanwhile, mix the dressing ingredients together with any remaining oil in the plastic bag.

4 Spoon the vegetables on to serving plates and drizzle the dressing over the top. Garnish with extra rosemary leaves torn from the stems.

NUTRITION

- Carbohydrate 3 g
- Fat 9 g
- Protein 5 g
- Energy 109 kcal (454 kJ)

Days 11 and 32

BREAKFAST

150 ml (¼ pint) glass of orange juice

Bowl of wholegrain cereal
Make with 75 g (3 oz) wholegrain cereal and 150 ml (¼ pint) skimmed or soya milk, adding 3 chopped dried apricots or prunes to sweeten.

OR

150 ml (¼ pint) glass of apple juice

2 boiled eggs and 1 slice of wholegrain bread spread thinly with olive oil spread

MID-MORNING SNACK

2 rice cakes spread thinly with low-fat cream cheese

LUNCH

Vegetable omelette
Make with 2 eggs and add chopped red pepper, spring onion and courgette.

OR

Mixed rice and vegetables
Mix 75 g (3 oz) cooked brown and wild rice with 125 g (4 oz) chopped grilled chicken and some chopped red pepper, spring onion and sweetcorn. Mix the juice of ½ lemon, 1 teaspoon olive oil and black pepper, and pour over the rice.

MID-AFTERNOON SNACK

Fruit smoothie
Blend together 1 kiwifruit, 1 sliced banana, 2 chopped dried apricots, 1 teaspoon honey and 250 ml (8 fl oz) skimmed or soya milk, then add 2 tablespoons low-fat natural yogurt.

TIP OF THE DAY

Keep a bowl of cherry tomatoes, sliced sweet peppers, and celery, carrot and cucumber sticks in the fridge, ready for those times when you feel the need to snack.

DINNER

Flaming chicken
Serves 4

Fry 4 chicken breasts, about 150 g (5 oz) each, and 200 g (7 oz) halved shallots in 1 tablespoon olive oil until the chicken is browned underneath. Turn it over and add 1 chopped garlic clove, 1 diced apple and 75 g (3 oz) sliced mushrooms. Fry until cooked. Spoon 4 tablespoons Calvados over the chicken and flame with a match. Once the flames subside, add 250 ml (8 fl oz) stock, 1 teaspoon mustard and thyme. Season and cook for 5 minutes. Serve with steamed vegetables.

OR

Vegetable noodles
Serves 4

Stir-fry 2 chopped peppers, 200 g (7 oz) each mangetout, sliced mushrooms and courgettes and 150 g (5 oz) baby sweetcorn in 2 tablespoons each soy sauce and olive oil for 5 minutes. Add 625 g (1¼ lb) buckwheat noodles and fry until cooked.

Oriental melon
(see recipe)

Oriental Melon

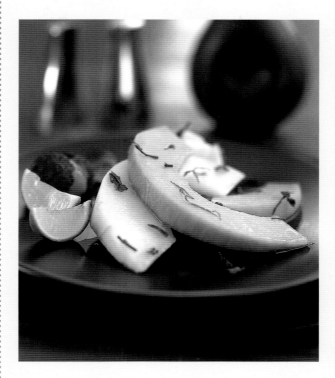

Preparation time: 15 minutes, plus chilling
Cooking time: none
Serves 6

2 orange-flavoured green teabags
300 ml (½ pint) boiling water
1 orange-fleshed cantaloupe melon, such as charentais
½ green-fleshed melon, such as galia or ogen
½ honeydew melon
2 tablespoons light cane sugar
grated rind and juice of 1 lime

To decorate
lime wedges
6 fresh lychees

1 Put the teabags into a jug and pour the boiling water over them. Leave to infuse for 2 minutes (no longer or it will taste bitter). Lift out the bags, draining them well. Break open one of the bags, remove a few tea leaves and add them to the tea infusion. Leave to cool.

2 Halve the whole melon and scoop out the seeds. Remove the seeds from the other melons. Cut away the skin with a small knife and cut the orange- and green-fleshed melons into long, thin slices. Dice the honeydew melon. Put all the prepared melon into a large, shallow dish.

3 Sprinkle the sugar and lime rind and juice over the melon and pour over the tea. Cover with clingfilm and chill for 1 hour, or overnight if preferred.

4 Arrange the long melon slices in fan shapes on individual serving plates. Spoon the diced melon to the side of the melon fans and serve each one with lime wedges and a partially peeled lychee.

NUTRITION

- Carbohydrate 20 g
- Fat 0 g
- Protein 2 g
- Energy 83 kcal (353 kJ)

Days 12 and 33

BREAKFAST

200 ml (7 fl oz) glass of pineapple juice

2 scrambled eggs and 1 slice of wholemeal toast spread thinly with olive oil spread

OR

200 ml (7 fl oz) glass of pomegranate juice

Bowl of muesli
Make with 75 g (3 oz) sugar-free muesli and 150 ml (¼ pt) skimmed or soya milk.

MID-MORNING SNACK

Pear and a small handful of pumpkin seeds

LUNCH

Tuna or feta salad
Make with 75 g (3 oz) fresh or 65 g (2½ oz) canned tuna or 50 g (2 oz) feta cheese and mixed salad leaves (baby spinach, watercress, lettuce), bean sprouts, 5 cherry tomatoes and fresh coriander and basil leaves. Dress with a little olive oil and cider vinegar

3 oatcakes

OR

Wholegrain turkey sandwich
Spread 2 slices wholegrain bread with 1 teaspoon low-calorie mayonnaise and fill with 150 g (5 oz) lean turkey breast, lettuce and sliced tomato.

Pieces of fruit
Choose from 2 kiwifruit, 2 plums or a pear.

MID-AFTERNOON SNACK

Plum and a small handful of almonds

DINNER

Scallops in pancetta with lemon lentils
(see recipe)

OR

Tempeh with lemon lentils
(see recipe)

Substitute the scallops and pancetta with tempeh for a vegetarian option.

150 g (5 oz) low-fat fruit yogurt per person

Scallops in Pancetta with Lemon Lentils

Preparation time: 15 minutes
Cooking time: 45 minutes
Serves 4

16 scallops, about 400 g (13 oz) in total, roe removed
2 tablespoons chopped oregano leaves
200 g (7 oz) pancetta, cut into 16 thin slices

Lemon lentils
1 teaspoon olive oil
1 onion, chopped
6 cloves
225 g (7½ oz) Puy lentils, washed
400 ml (14 fl oz) vegetable stock
400 ml (14 fl oz) hot water
4–6 tablespoons lemon juice
pepper

To garnish
mixed salad leaves
1 lemon, cut into 4 wedges
150 g (5 oz) low-fat Greek yogurt sprinkled with lemon zest
handful of oregano leaves

1 Prepare the lemon lentils by heating the olive oil in a saucepan over medium to low heat. Add the onion and cook for about 5 minutes, stirring occasionally, until it begins to brown. Add the whole cloves and lentils and cook for 5 minutes.

2 Pour in the vegetable stock and the measurement water and bring to the boil. Simmer gently, uncovered, for 30 minutes until the lentils are tender.

3 Meanwhile, sprinkle the scallops with the chopped oregano and wrap each in a slice of pancetta. Thread 4 scallop parcels on to a skewer. Repeat with the rest of the scallops. Grill the scallops on a barbecue or under a preheated hot grill for 2–3 minutes each side until they are golden brown.

4 Remove and discard the cloves from the lentils and stir in the lemon juice and pepper. Serve the scallops and lentils garnished with mixed salad leaves, a lemon wedge and yogurt, and sprinkled with oregano leaves.

NUTRITION

- Carbohydrate 36 g
- Fat 16 g
- Protein 47 g
- Energy 467 kcal (1967 kJ)

Days 13 and 34

BREAKFAST

150 ml (¼ pint) glass of tomato juice

Bowl of porridge
Make with 75 g (3 oz) rolled oats and 200 ml (7 fl oz) skimmed or soya milk, using 1 grated apple to sweeten.

OR

150 ml (¼ pint) glass of orange juice

Crunchy yogurt
Mix 1 tablespoon each toasted jumbo oats and mixed berries (strawberries, blueberries, blackberries, raspberries) into 150 g (5 oz) low-fat natural yogurt and sprinkle 2 tablespoons mixed seeds (pumpkin, sunflower, sesame) on top.

MID-MORNING SNACK

2 oatcakes spread thinly with peanut butter

LUNCH

Savoury bagel
Spread a bagel with 25 g (1 oz) low-fat cream cheese and top with 25 g (1 oz) smoked salmon.

OR

Wholemeal pitta with cottage cheese
Fill a pitta with 125 g (4 oz) cottage cheese, sliced cucumber and chopped chives.

Orange or mango

MID-AFTERNOON SNACK

Small handful of toasted nuts
Grill almonds, cashew nuts or walnuts, or a mixture of these, for 5–7 minutes.

TIP OF THE DAY

Make time to eat! You may have had a long day or need to rush off somewhere, but sitting down and really enjoying your food is important for both your digestive system and your health.

DINNER

**Marinated prawns
with courgettes**
(see recipe)

OR

Quinoa and rice fluff
Serves 4

Fry 1 chopped onion in
1 tablespoon olive oil until
soft, then add 125 g (4 oz)
each quinoa and brown
rice and 600 ml (1 pint)
vegetable stock, cover and
simmer until the stock has
been absorbed and the
rice is soft. Add salt and
pepper, juice of 1 lemon
and 1 tablespoon chopped
coriander.

Fresh pineapple
Allow 1 large slice (about
150 g/5 oz) per person.

Marinated Prawns with Courgettes

Preparation time:
30 minutes, plus marinating
Cooking time: 5 minutes
Serves 4

450 g (14½ oz) courgettes,
  topped and tailed and
  sliced into fine ribbons
  with a vegetable peeler
28 large raw prawns, peeled
  but with tails still intact,
  heads removed
handful of chopped flat-leaf
  parsley, to garnish

Marinade
large pinch of saffron
  threads
8 tablespoons lemon juice
6 garlic cloves, roughly
  chopped
2 tablespoons rice wine
  vinegar
4 tablespoons olive oil
2 tablespoons drained
  capers

1 Mix together all the marinade ingredients, lightly
crushing the capers against the side of the bowl.

2 Spoon two-thirds of the marinade mixture on top of the
courgette ribbons in a large bowl. Marinate for 3–4 hours.

3 Prepare the prawns. Hold the tail underside up and
cut each prawn in half lengthways. Pull out any black
intestinal thread, rinse, pat dry on kitchen paper and put
in a shallow dish. Alternatively, ask your fishmonger to
prepare the prawns for you. Pour the remaining marinade
over the prawns and marinate for 3–4 hours.

4 Place the courgettes in a large pan with their marinade
and simmer over a medium-low heat for 3–5 minutes.

5 Grill the prawns for 3–4 minutes until pink and sizzling,
basting with the marinade. Do not overcook them.

6 To serve, pile the courgettes in the centre of a warmed
dish, top with the prawns and garnish with chopped
parsley. Accompany with 75 g (3 oz) brown rice and
steamed broccoli with 1 teaspoon toasted sesame seeds.

NUTRITION

- Carbohydrate 6 g
- Fat 12 g
- Protein 12 g
- Energy 175 kcal/728 kJ

Days 14 and 35

BREAKFAST

150 ml (¼ pint) glass of pomegranate juice

2 large grilled tomatoes on 1 slice of wholegrain toast

OR

150 ml (¼ pint) glass of orange juice

Savoury omelette
Make with 2 eggs and chopped red pepper and mushrooms.

TIP OF THE DAY

Eggs are more effective for building muscle than any other protein – and more muscle means less body fat.

MID-MORNING SNACK

Pear

LUNCH

6 pieces of vegetarian sushi

Exotic fruit salad
Use chopped kiwifruit, pineapple, mango, passion fruit and papaya. Keep the remainder for your mid-afternoon snack.

OR

Vegetable and bean soup
Serves 6

Gently fry 2 onions, 1 celery stalk, 1 garlic clove and 550 g (1 lb 2 oz) mixed vegetables (carrots, green beans, broccoli), all chopped, with ½ teaspoon coriander seeds for about 5 minutes. Add 200 g (7 oz) chopped sweet potatoes, cover the pan and fry gently for 3–4 minutes, until soft. Add 1 litre (1¾ pints) vegetable stock, 400 g (13 oz) flageolet beans and 2 tablespoons chopped fresh herbs. Bring to the boil, then simmer for 10–15 minutes. The soup can be puréed before serving. Serve with a wholemeal roll, if required.

Pear, peach or nectarine

MID-AFTERNOON SNACK

Any fruit left over from your lunchtime fruit salad

OR

2 oatcakes and fruit
Choose from mango or peach, or 6 dried apricots or dates.

DINNER

Baked salmon fillet

Sprinkle a 150 g (5 oz) salmon fillet per person with lemon juice and pepper. Wrap in foil and bake in a preheated oven, 200°C (400°F), Gas Mark 6, for 12–15 minutes. Serve with sweet potato wedges, broccoli and carrots.

OR

Pasta with broccoli, olives and mozzarella
Serves 4

Cook 500 g (1 lb) broccoli florets until just tender and drain. Fry 1 chopped onion and 1 crushed garlic clove until soft. Add 400 g (13 oz) can chopped tomatoes, 1 tablespoon tomato purée, 125 g (4 oz) pitted black olives, the cooked broccoli and 2 tablespoons thyme. Cook for 3 minutes and season with salt and pepper. Cook 360 g (12³⁄₄ oz) wholemeal pasta, toss in the sauce and add 125 g (4 oz) low-fat buffalo mozzarella, torn into pieces. Serve with a tomato and basil salad.

Baked peaches
(see recipe)

Baked Peaches

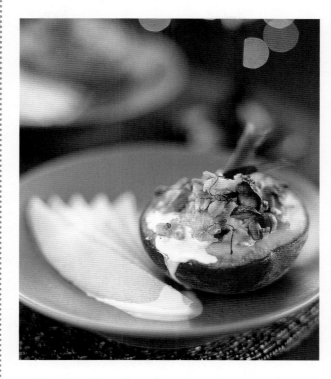

Preparation time:
15 minutes
Cooking time: 15 minutes
Serves 4

2 large, slightly under-ripe peaches, halved and pitted
a few saffron threads
a few drops almond extract
30 g (1¼ oz) crunchy oat cereal
2 tablespoons orange juice
5 cm (2 in) cinnamon stick, broken into 8 pieces

To serve
½ slightly under-ripe mango, thinly sliced
1 teaspoon grated dark chocolate (optional)

1 Scoop some of the flesh out of the peach halves and chop finely. Put the halved peaches, skin side down, in a lightly oiled baking dish.

2 Mix together the chopped peach flesh, saffron, almond extract, oat cereal and orange juice. Spoon the mixture carefully into the peach halves.

3 Push the cinnamon stick pieces into the peach halves. Bake the peaches uncovered in a preheated oven, 180°C (350°F), Gas Mark 4, for 15 minutes.

4 Arrange one peach half on each dessert plate. Serve with mango slices and a sprinkling of grated dark chocolate (if using).

NUTRITION

• Carbohydrate 16 g
• Fat 6 g
• Protein 3 g
• Energy 130 kcal (547 kJ)

Days 15 and 36

BREAKFAST

Fruit smoothie
Blend together 65 ml
(2½ fl oz) low-fat natural
yogurt and 75 g (3 oz) each
strawberries, blueberries
and raspberries. Add a few
pumpkin seeds and crushed
ice if liked.

OR

**150 ml (¼ pint) glass
of apple juice**

Bowl of muesli
Make with 75 g (3 oz) sugar-
free muesli and 200 ml
(7 fl oz) skimmed or soya
milk, using 1 sliced banana
to sweeten.

MID-MORNING SNACK

**Small handful of grapes
or 2 rice cakes lightly
spread with goat's
cheese and 2 cherry
tomatoes**

LUNCH

Cauliflower cheese soup
Serves 4

Fry 1 finely chopped onion in
1½ tablespoons olive oil
until soft. Add 750 g
(1½ lb) cauliflower florets,
cover and cook for 5–10
minutes. Stir in 600 ml
(1 pint) vegetable stock and
simmer until the cauliflower
is tender. Lightly toast some
pumpkin seeds. Purée the
soup, add 40 g (1½ oz)
grated strong Cheddar
cheese and salt and pepper.
Reheat until the cheese
melts. Garnish with a swirl
of fromage frais and the
toasted pumpkin seeds.
Serve with 1 slice of
wholegrain or rye bread.

OR

Chicken and rice salad
Mix 4 tablespoons cooked
brown rice with a large
handful of chopped raw
vegetables (cucumber,
celery, red pepper,
tomatoes, spring onions)
and 125 g (4 oz) chopped
grilled chicken. Squeeze
over 1 teaspoon lemon juice
and drizzle with 1 teaspoon
olive oil.

MID-AFTERNOON SNACK

**Vegetable crudités
with guacamole**
Make the guacamole by
mashing a ripe avocado into
the juice of 1 lime and
1 tablespoon soy sauce. For
the crudités, use a handful
of chopped, raw vegetables
(carrots, cucumber, peppers,
celery, cherry tomatoes).

TIP OF THE DAY

Focus on how you want to
look and keep that
picture in your mind —
this is what you are
working towards.

DINNER

Bean and lamb roast
(see recipe)

OR

Prawn stir-fry
Serves 2

Stir-fry 1 garlic clove and a 2.5 cm (1 in) piece fresh root ginger, both finely chopped, with 4 chopped spring onions and ½ teaspoon chilli powder for 2 minutes. Add 100 g (3½ oz) mangetout and sliced mushrooms and ½ sliced red pepper, and stir-fry for 4 minutes. Add 75 g (3 oz) shredded Chinese leaves, 100 g (3½ oz) bean sprouts, 200 g (7 oz) cooked jumbo prawns and 1 tablespoon light soy sauce, and heat gently.

Strawberries and yogurt
For each person, spoon 2 tablespoons low-fat natural yogurt over a handful of strawberries, then sprinkle with some toasted sesame and sunflower seeds.

Bean and Lamb Roast

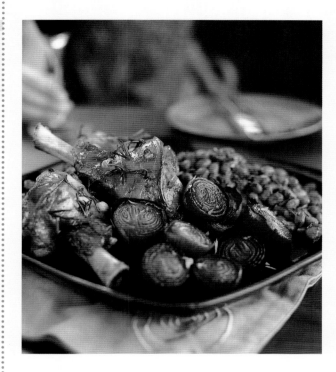

Preparation time:
10 minutes, plus marinating
Cooking time: 2–2½ hours
Serves 4

4 lamb shanks, about
  1.25 kg (2½ lb) in total,
  fat removed
4–5 rosemary sprigs
2 garlic cloves, thinly sliced
4 small red onions, halved
3 tablespoons balsamic
  vinegar

Marinade
**small bunch of thyme, leaves
  removed from stalks
3 whole cardamom pods
1 bay leaf
pinch of saffron threads
4 tablespoons lemon juice
salt and pepper**

Spiced beans
**2 teaspoons rapeseed oil
½ teaspoon black mustard
  seeds
½ teaspoon onion seeds
1 tablespoon tomato purée
pinch of ground turmeric
¼–½ teaspoon chilli powder
2 x 300 g (10 oz) cans pinto
  beans, drained
2 tablespoons chopped
  coriander leaves, plus
  extra to garnish**

1 Place the shanks in a roasting tin, make slits in each shank and push in sprigs of rosemary and slices of garlic.

2 Mix the marinade ingredients together. Coat the lamb shanks, cover with foil and refrigerate for at least 1 hour.

3 Cook the lamb in a preheated oven, 160°C (325°F), Gas Mark 3, for 2–2½ hours, basting every 45 minutes or so, until the meat is tender.

4 Meanwhile, prepare the beans. Heat the oil and cook the mustard and onion seeds over a low heat, letting them pop for a few seconds. Stir in the tomato purée, turmeric and chilli powder. Add the beans and a few tablespoons of hot water. Cover and cook for a few minutes. Stir in the chopped coriander leaves and remove from the heat.

5 Preheat the grill. Place the halved onions, cut sides up, in a heatproof dish, pour over the vinegar and cook under a preheated medium grill for about 20 minutes until soft.

6 Serve with the spiced beans and grilled red onions and sprinkled with chopped coriander leaves. Accompany with steamed green vegetables (cabbage, spinach, kale).

NUTRITION

- Carbohydrate 10 g
- Fat 14 g
- Protein 33 g
- Energy 293 kcal (1230 kJ)

Days 16 and 37

BREAKFAST

150 ml (¼ pint) glass of pomegranate juice

Poached egg on 1 slice of rye or wholemeal bread

OR

150 ml (¼ pint) glass of grapefruit juice

Bowl of wholegrain cereal
Make with 75 g (3 oz) wholegrain cereal and 150 ml (¼ pint) skimmed or soya milk.

MID-MORNING SNACK

1 peach or 3 plums

LUNCH

Griddled aubergines with chilli toasts
(see recipe)

OR

Avocado open sandwich
Make with 1 slice of wholegrain bread, topped with sliced avocado and tomato, seasoned with pepper and drizzled with a little olive oil.

Nectarine or peach and 150 g (5 oz) low-fat fruit yogurt per person

MID-AFTERNOON SNACK

Small handful of nuts and seeds
Choose from Brazil nuts, pine nuts, almonds, sunflower seeds and pumpkin seeds.

TIP OF THE DAY

Three or more daily servings of wholegrains can reduce your risk of heart disease, certain cancers and Type 2 diabetes by up to 30 per cent.

Griddled Aubergines with Chilli Toasts

DINNER

Cod and roasted vegetables

Place 150 g (5 oz) cod and 50 g (2 oz) total sliced green pepper, courgette, fennel, fresh root ginger, garlic, artichoke and sweet potato per person with 1 chopped onion in a dish. Drizzle with 2 tablespoons olive oil and season with salt and pepper. Bake for 30 minutes in a preheated oven, 180°C (350°F), Gas Mark 4.

OR

Tofu and roasted vegetables

Prepare and cook exactly as above, substituting the cod with tofu.

Baked apples

Sprinkle 1 cooking apple per person with 1 teaspoon brown sugar, a pinch of ground cinnamon and a few sultanas, add a little water and bake in a preheated oven, 160°C (325°F), Gas Mark 3, for about 1 hour, basting the apple skin until it turns golden brown.

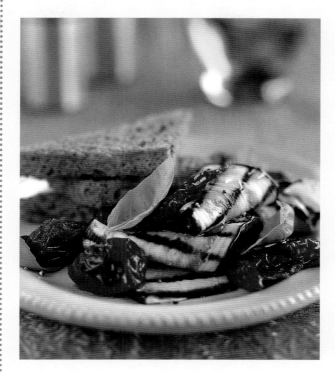

Preparation time: 15 minutes
Cooking time: 10 minutes
Serves 4

2 aubergines, about 550 g (1 lb 2 oz) in total
2 teaspoons olive oil
50 g (2 oz) sun-dried tomatoes
2 garlic cloves, crushed
4 tablespoons lemon juice

Chilli toasts
4 slices multigrain bread
1 tablespoon chilli-infused oil

To garnish
4 basil leaves
pepper

1 Prepare the chilli toasts. Remove the crusts from each slice of bread and cut the remaining bread into 2 neat triangles. Brush each side of the bread with chilli-infused oil and put the bread on an ovenproof baking sheet.

2 Cut the aubergines lengthways into 5 mm (¼ in) slices and season with pepper.

3 Put the chilli toasts in a preheated oven, 220°C (425°F), Gas Mark 7, and cook for 8–10 minutes until they are crisp and golden.

4 Meanwhile, oil a ridged griddle pan and heat it. Put the aubergine slices and sun-dried tomatoes on the pan with the garlic and cook for about 4 minutes until they start to soften. Turn over the aubergines and cook for a further 4 minutes. Finally, add the lemon juice.

5 Remove the chilli toasts from the oven and serve with the aubergine and tomato piled high in the centre of each plate and garnished with basil leaves and pepper.

NUTRITION

- Carbohydrate 15 g
- Fat 6 g
- Protein 4 g
- Energy 122 kcal (513 kJ)

Days 17 and 38

BREAKFAST

Fruit smoothie
Blend ½ mango and 1 banana with 150 ml (¼ pint) skimmed or soya milk and 100 ml (3½ fl oz) apple juice, then sprinkle with a few pumpkin seeds.

OR

150 ml (¼ pint) glass of apple juice

Bowl of porridge
Make with 75 g (3 oz) rolled oats and 200 ml (7 fl oz) skimmed or soya milk, and top with a few blueberries.

MID-MORNING SNACK

Small handful of white grapes or an apple

LUNCH

½ 400 g (13 oz) can vegetable soup and 1 slice of wholegrain or rye bread

OR

Cottage cheese and herb sandwich
Sandwich 2 slices rye or wholemeal bread with 50 g (2 oz) cottage cheese and chopped spring onions and fresh herbs (coriander, parsley, chives).

Apple

MID-AFTERNOON SNACK

2 oatcakes topped with 1 teaspoon hummus

TIP OF THE DAY

Are you hungry? Think about this really hard before you find yourself reaching for a snack: perhaps a glass of water would help, or call a friend for a chat.

DINNER

Spiced chicken and pearl barley
(see recipe)

OR

Vegetarian chilli
Serves 4

Sauté 1 chopped onion,
3 crushed garlic cloves and
½ teaspoon chilli powder in
30 ml (1¼ fl oz) vegetable
stock. Add 1 tablespoon
each tomato purée and
paprika and cook for 1
minute. Add a drained
400 g (13 oz) can each red
kidney beans and butter
beans and 500 g (1 lb) total
sliced carrots, courgettes,
peppers, mushrooms and
cauliflower. Simmer until the
vegetables are soft. Serve
with 1 wholemeal pitta
per person.

Fresh pineapple
Use 1 large slice (about
150 g/5 oz) per person.

Spiced Chicken and Pearl Barley

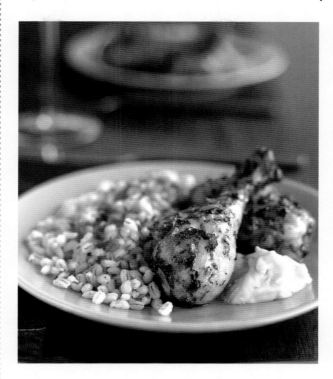

1 Combine all the ingredients for the spice mix in a bowl.
Rub the spice mix all over the chicken flesh. Set the
chicken aside for at least 2 hours to absorb the flavours.

2 Prepare the pearl barley. Heat the oil in a large, heavy-
based frying pan and cook the onion gently until soft,
stirring so it does not brown. Add the washed barley and
cook for 2 minutes. Pour in the stock and simmer for
1 hour, stirring occasionally, until all the fluid has been
absorbed and the grains are soft.

3 Meanwhile, cook the chicken, uncovered, in a preheated
oven, 190°C (375°F), Gas Mark 5, for 30–40 minutes until
it is tender throughout.

4 Make the raita. Combine the yogurt and grated
cucumber and sprinkle some cumin on the top.

5 When the chicken and pearl barley are cooked, garnish
the chicken with chopped parsley and serve immediately
with the pearl barley and raita. Accompany with mixed
salad leaves (endive, rocket, lamb's lettuce).

Preparation time:
45 minutes, plus marinating
Cooking time: 1 hour
Serves 4

1 kg (2 lb) chicken pieces on
the bone, skin removed
chopped parsley, to garnish

Spice mix
1 large onion, finely chopped
2 garlic cloves, chopped
½ teaspoon ground cumin
¼ teaspoon paprika
¼–½ teaspoon crushed
dried chillies
1–2 pinches saffron threads
6 tablespoons finely
chopped coriander
6 tablespoons finely
chopped flat-leaf parsley
2 tablespoons olive oil
2 tablespoons lemon juice

Pearl barley
1 teaspoon vegetable oil
1 small onion, chopped
200 g (7 oz) pearl barley
900 ml (1½ pints) chicken
stock

Raita
150 g (5 oz) low-fat natural
yogurt
125 g (4 oz) cucumber, grated
pinch of ground cumin

NUTRITION

- Carbohydrate 52 g
- Fat 13 g
- Protein 30 g
- Energy 428 kcal (1800 kJ)

Days 18 and 39

BREAKFAST

Small glass of tomato juice

Bowl of muesli
Make with 75 g (3 oz) sugar-free muesli and 150 ml (¼ pint) skimmed or soya milk, topped with a small handful of raspberries.

OR

150 ml (¼ pint) glass of pineapple juice

Ham and mushroom omelette
Make with 2 eggs, a few mushrooms and 1 oz (25 g) chopped lean ham.

MID-MORNING SNACK

Apple or banana

LUNCH

Spicy vegetable roast (see recipe)

OR

Cottage cheese and salad
Season 4 oz (125 g) cottage cheese with paprika and serve with mixed salad leaves (rocket, baby spinach, radicchio), topped with 6 cherry tomatoes and dressed with 1 teaspoon olive oil mixed with lemon juice.

MID-AFTERNOON SNACK

2 rice cakes spread thinly with peanut butter

TIP OF THE DAY

Berries are packed with fibre, so they will keep you feeling fuller for longer. They also contain powerful cancer-fighting antioxidants.

DINNER

Ginger baked chicken
Serves 4

Marinate 4 skinless chicken breasts (5 oz/150 g each) overnight in 1 cm (½ in) grated fresh root ginger, 1 crushed garlic clove, 2 chopped lemon slices, 3 tablespoons soy sauce and 4 tablespoons unsweetened apple juice. Cover with foil and bake in a preheated oven, 200°C (400°F), Gas Mark 6, for 30–40 minutes. Serve with spinach and boiled new potatoes.

OR

Tofu with vegetables
Serves 4

Sprinkle 375 g (12 oz) courgette and 250 g (8 oz) aubergine, cut into chunks, 225 g (7½ oz) halved tomatoes, 1 red pepper, 1 yellow pepper and 1 onion, all quartered, and 6 cloves garlic with 5 tablespoons olive oil and salt and pepper. Roast in a preheated oven, 200°C (400°F), Gas Mark 6, for 45 minutes. Serve with 125 g (4 oz) baked tofu per person.

Apple or pear per person

Spicy Vegetable Roast

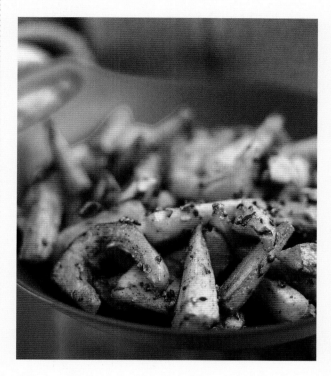

Preparation time:
15 minutes
Cooking time:
35–40 minutes
Serves 6

1 teaspoon fennel seeds
1 teaspoon cumin seeds
1 teaspoon coriander seeds
½ teaspoon turmeric
½ teaspoon paprika
2 garlic cloves, chopped
3 tablespoons olive oil
500 g (1 lb) butternut squash, peeled, halved, deseeded and thickly sliced
4 small parsnips, about 425 g (14 oz) in total, cut into quarters
3 carrots, about 300 g (10 oz) in total, cut into thick strips
salt and pepper

1 Crush the seeds using a pestle and mortar or use the end of a rolling pin. Transfer to a large plastic bag and add the turmeric, paprika, garlic, oil and salt and pepper. Squeeze the bag to mix the contents together.

2 Add the vegetables to the plastic bag, grip the top edge to seal and toss together until the vegetables are coated with the spices.

3 Tip the vegetables into a roasting tin and bake in a preheated oven, 200°C (400°F), Gas Mark 6, for 35–40 minutes, turning once until browned and tender. Transfer to a serving dish.

NUTRITION

- Carbohydrate 20 g
- Fat 7 g
- Protein 3 g
- Energy 147 kcal (619 kJ)

Days 19 and 40

BREAKFAST

Small glass of pomegranate juice

Bowl of porridge
Make with 75 g (3 oz) rolled oats and 200 ml (7 fl oz) skimmed or soya milk.

OR

150 ml (¼ pint) glass of apple juice

Poached egg on 1 slice of wholegrain bread

MID-MORNING SNACK

Orange or pear

LUNCH

Avocado and sunflower seed salad
Arrange avocado slices and a sprinkling of sunflower seeds on mixed salad leaves (radicchio, lamb's lettuce, watercress) with 6 cherry tomatoes and sliced cucumber. Drizzle with a dressing of 1 teaspoon each olive oil, white wine vinegar and lemon juice per person.

OR

Prawn tortilla
Fill a flour tortilla with 75 g (3 oz) prawns (or chicken), chopped tomatoes, cucumber and red pepper, mixed with 2 tablespoons low-fat natural yogurt, a squeeze of lemon juice and chopped chilli (optional). (Substitute the flour tortilla with 2 slices of wholegrain bread if preferred.)

Small bowl of strawberries

MID-AFTERNOON SNACK

Small handful of mixed nuts
Choose from walnuts, almonds, Brazil nuts or pine nuts.

TIP OF THE DAY

If you are working, prepare your lunch the night before and take it with you.

Almondy Angel Cakes

DINNER

Monkfish with asparagus
Serves 4

Mix 2 crushed garlic cloves, 1 teaspoon shredded fresh root ginger, 2 tablespoons soy sauce and ¼ teaspoon rice vinegar, and pour over 600 g (1¼ lb) boned, cubed monkfish tail. Cover the dish. Drizzle 200 g (7 oz) asparagus with olive oil. Roast fish and asparagus in a preheated oven, 200°C (400°F), Gas Mark 6, for 15–20 minutes. Serve with a leafy green vegetable.

OR

Bean and feta stir-fry
Serves 4

Fry 2–3 chopped garlic cloves and 1 chopped onion in 1 tablespoon olive oil. Add 3 chopped tomatoes, a drained 400 g (13 oz) can each red kidney and flageolet beans, 25 g (1 oz) black olives and 1 tablespoon soy sauce and lemon juice. Cook for 4–5 minutes. Add 100 g (3½ oz) feta cheese and season with fresh herbs and pepper.

Almondy angel cakes
(see recipe)

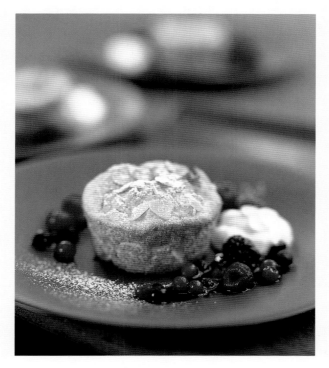

Preparation time:
15 minutes
Cooking time: 10–15 minutes
Serves 6

4 egg whites
1½ tablespoons caster sugar
50 g (2 oz) ground almonds
generous pinch of cream
   of tartar
15 g (½ oz) flaked almonds
400 g (13 oz) frozen mixed
   berry fruits
200 g (7 oz) fromage frais

1 Lightly oil 6 sections of a deep muffin tin and line the bases with circles of greaseproof paper.

2 Whisk the egg whites until stiff, moist peaks form. Whisk in the sugar, a teaspoonful at a time, until it has all been added and continue to whisk for a minute or two until the mixture is thick and glossy.

3 Fold in the ground almonds and cream of tartar and spoon the mixture into the sections of the muffin tin. Sprinkle the flaked almonds over the tops.

4 Cook in a preheated oven, 180°C (350°F), Gas Mark 4, for 10–12 minutes until golden brown and set. Loosen the edges of the cakes with a knife and lift them on to a cooling rack.

5 Warm the fruits in a saucepan. Arrange the angel cakes on serving plates, add a spoonful of fromage frais to each and spoon the fruits around.

NUTRITION

- Carbohydrate 8 g
- Fat 9 g
- Protein 7 g
- Energy 140 kcal (583 kJ)

Days 20 and 41

BREAKFAST

150 ml (¼ pint) glass of apple and mango juice

2 large grilled tomatoes on 1 slice of wholegrain toast spread thinly with olive oil spread

OR

200 ml (7 fl oz) glass of pomegranate juice

Crunchy yogurt
Mix 1 tablespoon each toasted jumbo oats and mixed berries (strawberries, blueberries, blackberries and raspberries) into 150 g (5 oz) low-fat natural yogurt and sprinkle sesame and sunflower seeds on top.

MID-MORNING SNACK

Peach or nectarine and 3 fresh or dried apricots

LUNCH

Hot chicken liver salad (see recipe)

OR

Rice salad
Serves 4

Mix together juice of 1 lemon, 1 crushed garlic clove, 1 tablespoon olive oil and salt and pepper. Stir the following into 50 g (2 oz) each cooked brown rice and cooked millet: 1 chopped bunch spring onions, 2 diced peppers, 2 chopped large tomatoes, ½ chopped cucumber, 50 g (2 oz) chopped mixed nuts (walnuts, almonds, Brazil nuts). Then pour the dressing over the top. Leave in the refrigerator to chill.

MID-AFTERNOON SNACK

2 rice cakes, spread thinly with tahini or topped with 2 tablespoons cottage cheese

TIP OF THE DAY

Oats are complex carbohydrates that release energy slowly, so you feel fuller for longer. They also help to stabilize blood sugar, discouraging you from snacking.

DINNER

Baked trout
Serves 4

Sprinkle 1 trout fillet (600 g/ 1¼ lb) with chopped dill and spring onions, lemon pepper and salt. Cover with foil and bake in a preheated oven, 200°C (400°F), Gas Mark 6, for 15–20 minutes. Garnish with toasted pine nuts and orange slices and serve with courgettes, spinach and carrots.

OR

Vegetable penne
Serves 4

Fry 1 chopped onion and 1 chopped garlic clove in 2 tablespoons olive oil until soft. Add a 200 g (7 oz) can tomatoes, 1 tablespoon each tomato pureé and lemon juice, and salt and pepper. Simmer for 10–15 minutes. Stir in 100 g (3½ oz) each torn spinach and sliced courgettes, 50 g (2 oz) baby sweetcorn, 2 tablespoons fresh herbs. Simmer for 2 minutes. Serve with 360 g (12¾ oz) wholemeal pasta.

Baked bananas
(see recipe on page 39)

Hot Chicken Liver Salad

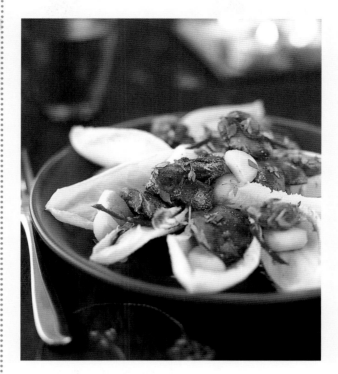

Preparation time:
5 minutes, plus soaking
Cooking time: 5 minutes
Serves 4

400 g (13 oz) chicken livers, trimmed and halved
60 ml (2½ fl oz) milk
2 teaspoons chopped thyme
1 tablespoon olive oil
2 garlic cloves, crushed
1 red chilli pepper, sliced thinly (optional)
200 g (7 oz) can water chestnuts, drained and halved

To serve
200 g (7 oz) chicory, leaves separated
1½–2 tablespoons balsamic vinegar

1 Soak the liver in milk for 30 minutes to remove any bitterness. Discard the milk and pat the liver dry with kitchen paper. Sprinkle the thyme over both sides of the liver.

2 Heat the oil in a large frying pan and add the garlic and sliced chilli (if using). Allow the garlic and chilli to soften for 30 seconds, then add the chicken livers and water chestnuts.

3 Cook over a medium heat for 3–4 minutes, until the liver is browned on the outside but still pink in the middle.

4 Serve on a bed of crispy raw chicory, drizzled with balsamic vinegar and any remaining pan juices.

NUTRITION

- Carbohydrate 9 g
- Fat 10 g
- Protein 21 g
- Energy 199 kcal (835 kJ)

Days 21 and 42

BREAKFAST

Banana smoothie
Blend together 1 banana,
150 ml (¼ pint) skimmed
milk and 150 g (5 oz) low-fat
natural yogurt, then sprinkle
with sunflower seeds.

OR

**150 ml (¼ pint) glass
of orange juice**

Bowl of porridge
Make with 75 g (3 oz) millet
or rolled oats and 200 ml
(7 fl oz) of skimmed or
soya milk, sprinkled with
flax seeds.

MID-MORNING SNACK

Apple or pear

LUNCH

Savoury omelette
Make with 2 eggs, chopped
mushrooms, red pepper and
onion, and serve with mixed
salad leaves (watercress,
rocket, lamb's lettuce).

OR

Tuna salad
Drain a 185 g (6½ oz)
can tuna and mix with
1 teaspoon olive oil and juice
of ½ lemon, chopped spring
onions and chives. Serve
the tuna on a bed of
mixed salad leaves (endive,
lettuce, baby spinach) with
6 cherry tomatoes.

MID-AFTERNOON SNACK

**Handful of grapes or
2 plums**

TIP OF THE DAY

The spice in peppers –
capsaicin – speeds up
your metabolism, helping
you to burn fat.

DINNER

Plaice parcels
(see recipe)

OR

Steak and mixed rice
Fry 1 chopped onion in 1 tablespoon olive oil until brown. Add 200 g (7 oz) wild rice and 500 ml (17 fl oz) vegetable stock and simmer until the stock has been absorbed. Meanwhile, grill 150 g (5 oz) steak per person. Serve with the rice and steamed vegetables.

Mango sorbet
Serves 6

Boil 50 g (2 oz) light cane sugar in 200 ml (7 fl oz) water until dissolved, then cool. Stir in the puréed flesh of 1 mango and juice of 500 g (1 lb) clementines and freeze in a plastic box for 2–3 hours until semi-frozen. Beat well, then freeze and beat again. Mix in 1 egg white and freeze until solid. Slice 1 mango and toss in the grated rind and juice of 1 lime. Soften the sorbet at room temperature for 15 minutes and serve with the mango slices.

Plaice Parcels

Preparation time:
30 minutes
Cooking time: 10 minutes
Serves 4

1 fennel bulb, about 360 g (11½ oz)
2 red chillies, deseeded and chopped
4 tablespoons lemon juice
2 teaspoons olive oil
4 plaice fillets, about 650 g (1 lb 6 oz) in total
1 small handful chopped dill
½ lemon, cut into wedges, to garnish

Radicchio and orange salad
200 g (7 oz) red radicchio leaves
2 large oranges, peeled and pith removed, separated into segments

1 Finely chop the fennel bulb and put it in a bowl with the chopped chillies. Add the lemon juice and olive oil to the fennel and set aside.

2 Cut 4 sheets of baking parchment, each 35 x 18 cm (14 x 7 in), and fold them in half widthways. Lay ½ sheet over a plate and arrange a fish fillet on one side of the fold. Sprinkle over some chopped dill and fold over the paper to enclose the filling. Fold in the edges and pleat to secure. Repeat with the remaining fish.

3 Place the wrapped fish on a baking sheet and cook in a preheated oven, 220°C (425°F), Gas Mark 7, for about 8 minutes or until the paper is puffed up and brown.

4 Make the salad by combining the radicchio with the orange segments.

5 Place each fish parcel on a large plate and cut an X-shaped slit in the top and curl back the paper, or pull the paper apart to open the parcel, releasing a fragrant puff of steam. Serve with individual side bowls of the fennel and chilli mixture and radicchio and orange salad, and garnish with a lemon wedge.

NUTRITION

- Carbohydrate 13 g
- Fat 6 g
- Protein 32 g
- Energy 234 kcal (988 kJ)

THE WAISTLINE

|1| |2| |3| |4| |5| |6| |7| |8| |9| |10| |11| |12| |13

EXERCISE PLAN

14 15 16 17 18 19 20 21 22 23 24 25 26

HOW THE EXERCISE PLAN WORKS

The Waistline Diet Plan will enable you to lose weight and feel healthier and more energized. At the same time, you can tone and flatten your stomach, and sculpt your hips, thighs and buttocks, by following the Waistline Exercise Plan. The combination of toning workouts and aerobic exercise will not only give you a new shape, it will also help you to achieve a new sense of confidence and wellbeing.

WHAT WILL IT DO FOR ME?

Exercise brings so many different benefits. Not only does it make you healthier and less stressed, it also makes you look and feel great and it even helps you to lose weight by speeding up your metabolism and enabling your body to burn fat for longer. Some people worry that they are too busy to commit to regular exercise or even that they are too unfit to begin. The Waistline Exercise Plan is all about showing how easy it is to bring regular exercise into your life, with short but effective sessions that can be fitted into your daily schedule without taking up too much of your time.

The Waistline Exercise Plan works by combining specific toning exercises that focus on the muscles of the stomach, hips, thighs and buttocks with an aerobic 'interval' exercise session that targets your heart and lungs, helping you to build strength and stamina and burn fat. It is this combination of aerobic and toning exercise that will help you to achieve a flatter, thinner you, which is why you must incorporate both sets of activities into your Plan – so don't forget to do one weekly aerobic session at the very least.

WHO IS IT FOR?

This exercise regime is suitable for everyone, from absolute beginners to those who exercise regularly. The Waistline Exercise Plan can be adapted to take into account your own specific exercise needs, so long as you achieve the minimum level of toning and exercise activity. Once you begin to exercise you will soon see the benefits. The more you exercise, the more energy you will have and the more you will want to exercise.

Continuing to use the Waistline Exercise Plan on a regular basis will mean you can maintain a healthy body-fat level in the future.

HOW MUCH SHOULD I DO?

To get real benefit from the Waistline Exercise Plan, you should do the toning exercises for 10 minutes per session (excluding warm-up and cool-down exercises), 3 times a day, 5 times a week. Along with these, you also need to include a 20-minute aerobic session each week. If you find this too much at first, begin with just 10 minutes of exercises per day, 5 days a week, along with your 20-minute aerobic session – but bear in mind that the results will be slower. You can then increase the duration and frequency of your exercise and aerobic sessions, building up to 30 minutes total of toning exercises, 5 days a week and 2 or more aerobic sessions. You must have 2 rest days per week, but that doesn't rule out a brisk walk or short swim on these days.

AEROBIC EXERCISES

- Brisk walking
- Jogging
- Skipping
- Step
- Dancing
- Swimming
- Cycling
- Rowing
- Netball
- Tennis
- Squash
- Hockey
- Basketball
- Rollerblading

IMPORTANT MUSCLES

1 **Biceps** – front of the upper arm, used to move the arm.

2 **Triceps** – back of the upper arm, used to move the arm.

3 **Deltoid** – encloses the shoulder and upper arm, used to move the arm backwards and forwards.

4 **Trapezius** – runs down the back of the neck and along the shoulders, used to extend the head.

5 **Rhomboid** – attaches the shoulder blades to the spine. Mostly lies beneath the trapezius muscle.

6 **Latissimus dorsi** – popularly referred to as 'lats', it runs from the lower chest into the lumbar region. It pulls the shoulders down and back and the body upwards.

7 **Erector spinae** – (not shown) found at the back of the neck, chest and abdomen. This important muscle extends the spine and holds the body upright.

8 **Quadratus lumborum** – (not shown) deep interior waist muscle. It bends the torso sideways.

9 **Transversus abdominis** – (not shown) deep internal muscle that runs across the abdomen. It applies pressure to the abdomen and holds the organs in place. It lies beneath the internal oblique muscle (see 10).

10 **Internal oblique** – (not shown) horizontally crosses the abdomen, compresses the abdomen and moves the trunk. It lies beneath the external oblique muscle (see 11).

11 **External oblique** – side muscle of the abdomen. It compresses the abdomen and is used when moving the trunk in any direction.

12 **Rectus abdominis** – popularly known as the 'abs', this muscle runs vertically down the entire front of the abdomen. This postural muscle draws the front of the pelvis upwards.

13 **Perineum** – (not shown) an internal muscle. It forms the pelvic floor and attaches to the pelvic wall, which is located deep in the pelvic cavity.

14 **Psoas** – (not shown) this deep muscle is part of the hip flexor. It runs from the front of the femur to the lumbar region of the spine. It acts to bring the thigh forwards at the hip.

15 **Adductor** – an inner thigh muscle, used for moving the leg inward.

16 **Gluteus maximus** – forms the buttocks. It is used for walking, running and jumping.

17 **Quadriceps extensor** – runs down the middle of the front of the thigh. It performs the opposite movement to the semitendinosus or hamstrings.

18 **Semitendinosus** – also known as the hamstrings. This muscle runs down the middle of the back of the thigh. Used to extend the thigh and to flex the leg at the knee joint.

19 **Gastrocnemius** – this muscle runs down the back of the lower leg and forms the greater part of the calf. It gives the force when walking and running.

20 MINUTES OF AEROBIC EXERCISE

Aerobic exercise requires the use of oxygen and involves the lungs, heart and blood circulation system of the body. It helps to burn calories, reduces stress levels and the production of cortisol, lowers blood pressure, develops cardiovascular fitness and improves your cholesterol levels. Once you find your session easy, or you wish to lose weight more quickly, you can build more sessions into your week.

During your 20-minute 'interval' exercise session, you should alternate bouts of short, sharp, intense activity with short periods of lower intensity activity. This method of exercising has been shown to promote weight loss. For example, if you are jogging you would warm up for 5 minutes, then run hard and fast for 1–2 minutes (depending on your fitness level), then jog to

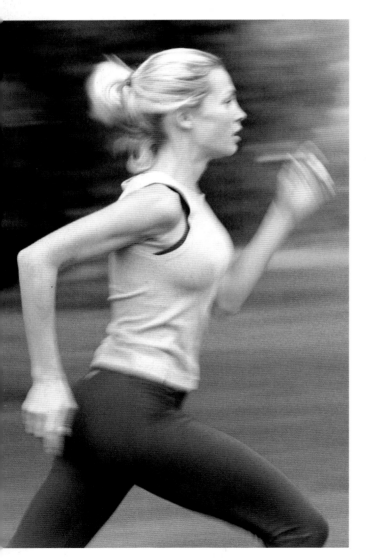

recover for another 2 minutes. You would then simply repeat the process for 20 minutes. This method can be applied to all the aerobic exercise suggestions (see panel on page 72).

If you find it difficult to exercise for the full 20 minutes to begin with, gradually build yourself up to it. You can choose a mix of several aerobic exercises if you prefer: for example, running and rowing, or cycling, stepping and dancing. To avoid stiffness or injury, make sure you remember both to warm up and cool down thoroughly both before and after any aerobic session (see below).

PUTTING IT ALL TOGETHER

Before you begin an exercise session, you need to make sure your muscles are thoroughly warmed up. Try brisk walking, jogging on the spot, gentle or stationary cycling, rowing, stepping or skipping for around 5 minutes. You should feel warm but not exhausted.

- Move on to the warm-up stretches on pages 77–83. These are important, so do not miss them out.
- Now select at least 3 exercises from pages 84–95 (for the buttocks, hips and thighs) and 5 from pages 96–117 (for the stomach).
- Follow these with the cool-down stretches on pages 118–123. To cool down, you can also use some of the warm-up stretches on pages 77–83.

Reps and sets

Each exercise specifies the number of reps (repetitions) and sets you should perform. Reps are the number of times you repeat an exercise in one go, while a set is the completed number of repetitions. So, if you perform 3 sets of 8 reps each, you will perform 24 repetitions of the exercise in all.

For exercises performed on both sides of the body, the number of reps specified is for one side only.

USING HAND WEIGHTS

When you start to feel fitter and stronger, use small hand weights to increase the resistance training effect of the following exercises:

- **Knee lifts** (see page 83)
- **Squats** (see page 84)
- **Arabesque** (see page 90)
- **Lunges with lateral raises** (see page 92)

Work those muscles!

At the start of each exercise, you will be told which muscles are being targeted. Unless you already know which muscles are which, you will probably find it useful to refer to the diagrams and explanations on page 73, which describe where the important muscles in the body are and what they do.

SAMPLE WORKOUT ROUTINE

Warm-up

- Upper body warm-up (see page 77)
- Side stretch (see page 78)
- Side twist (see page 79)
- Calf stretch (see page 80)
- Hamstring stretch (see page 81)
- Quads stretch (see page 82)
- Knee lifts (see page 83)

Toning exercises

- Squats (see page 84)
- Buttock kicks (see page 86)
- Bottom lifts (see page 87)
- Leg lifts (see page 88)
- Lunges with lateral raises (see page 92)
- Inner thigh lifts (see page 94)
- Roll-ups (see page 96)
- Scissors (see page 102)
- The plank (see page 104)
- Tummy tighteners (see page 108)
- Oblique crunch (see page 110)

Cool-down

- Groin stretch (see page 118)
- Inner thigh stretch (see page 119)
- Spinal twist (see page 120)
- Pose of the child (see page 122)

COMFORT AND SAFETY

Wear appropriate clothing for your workout. Anything comfortable such as a T-shirt and leggings or shorts is fine, and for women a sports bra is a good investment. You will need a suitable pair of trainers to act as shock absorbers and protect your feet. A towel or floor mat will also be useful to help protect your knees, hips and back.

It is important that you do not become dehydrated: drink water before, during and after exercise. Water keeps your body hydrated, flushes out toxins, repairs cells and helps to keep your skin looking good. Mineral or filtered water is best.

Steps

• REPS 5–10 MINS

Before you begin exercising, warm up the body with some gentle aerobic exercise, such as jogging on the spot, skipping or stepping, then follow with some of the warm-up stretches on pages 77–83.

Step on and off a step alternately with each foot.

Upper body warm-up

• **REPS 10**
• **SETS 1–2**

These upper body warm-up exercises are good for opening the chest, stretching the pectoral muscles and lengthening the spine.

WATCHPOINTS

- As you circle, keep your back long and straight and your shoulders down

- Stretch your arms and fingers straight up, palms facing in

- Keep your stomach pulled in

1

2

Stand with your feet facing forwards and hip-width apart, your stomach pulled in and your arms hanging loosely at your sides. Circle your arms forwards and around. Repeat in a backwards circular motion.

Cross your right arm in front of your body. Place your left hand on your right upper arm and press firmly. Hold for a count of 10, then repeat with your other arm.

Side stretch

- **REPS 5–8**
- **SETS 1**

This exercise will stretch and tone the external oblique muscles that run down the sides of your waist. You will soon find that your hand can reach down past your knee.

WATCHPOINTS

- Try to keep your stomach pulled in
- Breathe out on the way down and in on the way up
- Allow your head to drop right over to your shoulder as you stretch

Stand with your feet facing forwards and hip-width apart, with your arms hanging loosely at your sides.

Exhale and slide your right arm down your right side, letting your shoulders and head drop to the right, and stretching your fingers downward. Make sure you pull in your stomach to maximize the stretch. Inhale and return to the starting position. Repeat on the left side.

Side twist

• **REPS** 10
• **SETS** 1

This is a great exercise for toning and tightening your waist, working on the external oblique muscles.

WATCHPOINTS

1 2 3 4 5 6 7 8 9 10 11 12 13

• Make sure your knees are slightly bent

• Remember to push your elbows back

• Keep your back long

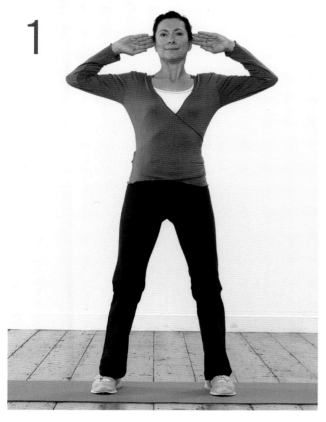

Stand with your feet facing forwards and slightly wider than hip-width apart. Place your hands each side of your head, elbows facing outward. Bend your knees slightly.

Twist your body to the right, pushing both elbows backward. Return to the starting position and then repeat to the left.

Calf stretch

- **REPS 3**
- **SETS 1–5**

This movement stretches the gastrocnemius or calf muscle. It can be used for both the warm-up and the cool-down.

WATCHPOINTS

- Hold on to a bar or push against the wall to make this movement easier
- Keep your toes pointing forward

1

Stand straight, with both feet together. Put your hands on your hips and lengthen your spine.

2

Step forwards with your left leg. Lean from the hips, placing your weight on a slightly bent left leg. Keep your right foot straight and flat on the floor and feel the stretch through your right calf. Hold for a count of 10. Return to the starting position and repeat with your left leg.

Hamstring stretch

• **REPS 3** • **SETS 1–2**

This stretch will lengthen the hamstrings, helping to prevent injury. It can be used for both the warm-up and the cool-down.

WATCHPOINTS

- **Push out your buttocks to feel the stretch.**
- **Keep your chest lifted**

1

Stand with both feet together. Extend your left leg in front of you, keeping the foot on the floor. Bend your right knee. Bend from the hips and feel the stretch through the back of your left leg.

2

Keeping your right foot on the floor, lift the toes of your left foot towards you. Keep the heel on the floor and feel the stretch through the back of your left leg. Hold for a count of 10. Return to the starting position and repeat with your right leg.

Quads stretch

• **REPS 3**
• **SETS 1–2**

This stretch works the quadriceps muscles of the thighs. It is an excellent exercise to incorporate in both your warm-up and cool-down routines.

WATCHPOINTS

- Push your hips slightly forward to increase the stretch.
- Keep your back long and straight
- If you find it difficult to keep your balance, use a chair or wall for support

Stand with your left hand either out in front or to the side to help you balance. Bend your right knee and take hold of the front of the foot with your right hand. Pull your right heel back towards your right buttock, keeping your knees in line with each other. You will feel a stretch down the front of your thigh. Hold for a count of 10. Repeat with your left leg.

Knee lifts

This warm-up exercise is good for toning your waist as it works the stomach muscles – the external obliques and the abdominals. It also strengthens the quadriceps muscles of the thighs.

• **REPS 10–16**
• **SETS 1–2**

WATCHPOINTS

- Keep your back straight and shoulders down

- Rotate around your waist in order to work the oblique muscles

Stand with your feet facing forwards and hip-width apart. Lift your right knee to chest height and take your left elbow across to your right knee. Repeat, lifting your left knee to chest height and taking your right elbow across to your left knee.

Variations

To introduce an aerobic element to this exercise, add a hop with each knee lift. To increase the intensity of the exercise, hold a hand weight in each hand.

Squats

This first exercise from the workout proper strengthens the quadriceps muscles in the thighs, the hamstrings, the gluteus medius on the hip and the gluteus maximus in the buttocks.

• REPS 10
• SETS 1–3

WATCHPOINTS

- Keep your feet flat on the floor
- Don't squat down too quickly
- Make sure your buttocks do not go any lower than your knees

1

Stand with your feet facing forwards and hip-width apart. Place your hands on your hips and pull in your stomach. Keeping your back straight, bend 90 degrees at the knees, leaning forwards until your body is at 90 degrees to your thighs. Keep your feet flat on the floor. Hold the position for a count of 3.

2

Using your thigh muscles, push back up to the starting position but do not straighten your legs completely before repeating. To increase the intensity of the exercise, add hand weights.

Squat jumps

This exercise works the quadriceps, hamstrings, gluteus medius and gluteus maximus muscles. It is more taxing than squats, and you may only manage 3 or 4 repetitions to begin with.

WATCHPOINTS

- Do only as many repetitions as you can to begin with
- Remember to bend your knees when you land
- Keep your chin and head up

1

Stand with your feet facing forwards and hip-width apart, your stomach pulled in and your hands on your hips. Squat down as before.

2

Now jump up. Tap your heels together in mid-air and land with your feet apart, back in the squat position.

Buttock kicks

This exercise works on toning the gluteus medius and gluteus maximus muscles of your hips and buttocks, as well as the hip flexors. It also strengthens the hamstrings.

WATCHPOINTS

• **Keep your stomach pulled up to your spine**

• **Push your leg as high as you can without strain**

• **Keep the exercise slow and controlled**

1

Kneel on all fours with your elbows under your chest and knees under your hips. Lower your body downwards, on to your elbows.

2

Lift your left leg off the floor, keeping your knee bent at 90 degrees, until the sole of your foot is facing the ceiling. Raise your foot high above your buttocks. Hold and squeeze your buttocks for 2 seconds. Lower your leg to the starting position and repeat with your right leg.

Bottom lifts

Strengthening the quadriceps muscles and the gluteus maximus and minimus muscles, this exercise tones your bottom. It also works the abdominal muscles and the lower back.

WATCHPOINTS

- Keep your bottom off the floor during the exercise
- Pull your stomach down and in tightly
- Curl up through your pelvis

Lie on your back with both knees bent and your feet flat on the floor, hip-width apart. Place your hands flat on the floor, with your arms at the sides of your body.

Raise your hips off the floor as far as you can. Lift and squeeze your buttocks together tightly. Hold for a count of 4, then lower your hips back down to the floor.

Leg lifts

This exercise is great for toning the legs, working the quadriceps and hamstrings. It also targets hip and buttock muscles – the gluteus maximus, minimus and medius muscles and the hip flexors.

WATCHPOINTS

- Don't bend the knee of the lifted leg
- Keep your head down on your forearms

1

Lie face down on the floor, with your forehead resting on your forearms.

2

Lift up your left leg, straight out behind you. Hold for a count of 3, then lower. Repeat with your right leg.

Side leg lifts

This exercise strengthens the gluteus maximus and gluteus medius muscles of the buttocks, as well as the hip flexors. You may find your legs ache to begin with, but this will ease.

- **REPS 16**
- **SETS 1–3**

WATCHPOINTS

- Keep your body in a straight line throughout

- To stop yourself rolling backwards, push your hips forward

- Don't allow the lift to become a continuous movement – remember to hold

1

Lie on your right side with your body in a straight line, your right elbow bent and your right hand supporting your head. Place your left hand on the floor in front of you, close to your body, for support. Keeping your hips facing forward, bend your right knee on the floor so your right foot faces backward.

2

Lift your left leg as high as you can. Hold for a count of 2, then lower. Aim to do 16 lifts, then repeat on the other side.

Arabesque

• **REPS 16**
• **SETS 1–3**

This exercise works lower body muscles, such as the quadriceps of the thighs and the gluteus maximus muscles of the buttocks. The hip flexors and the erector spinae of the back are also targeted.

Stand with your feet together and hands on your hips. Incline your body forwards slightly from the hips, keeping your back straight and head up. Stretch your right leg out straight behind you.

Lift your right leg as high as you can manage comfortably. Hold for a count of 2, then lower. Repeat with your left leg.

WATCHPOINTS

- Keep your back straight

- Make sure your hips face forward, to protect your back

- Hold on to the back of a chair if you need some support as you lift

Variation

To increase the intensity of this exercise, hold a 2 kg (4½ lb) hand weight in each hand.

As you raise your leg, lift the hand weights straight up above your shoulder and over your head (the weights will enable you to lift your leg higher). Hold for a count of 2, then lower. Repeat with your other leg.

Lunges with lateral raises

This exercise is great for strengthening the buttocks, thighs and calves. The gluteals, quadriceps, hamstrings and gastrocnemius are the muscles worked here.

1

Stand with your feet together. Hold a light hand weight in each hand resting by your sides, palms facing in.

2

Take a large step forwards with your left leg, keeping your stomach tight and your back straight.

WATCHPOINTS

- Don't allow your bent knee to touch the floor

- Your shoulders must be in line with your hips

- Place the weight on the heel of your front foot to work the buttock muscle

3

Bend both knees, until your right knee is close to the floor. Raise the hand weights up and out to the sides until your arms are parallel to the floor. Hold for a count of 2. Using your right thigh, push back up to the starting position. At the same time, lower your arms back down to your sides. Repeat with your left leg.

Inner thigh lifts

This exercise specifically targets the hip adductor muscles of the inner thigh. You will need to keep your inner thigh tight throughout the exercise in order to work these muscles properly.

Lie on your right side with your body in a straight line, your right elbow bent and your right hand supporting your head. Place your left hand in front of you, close to your body, for support.

Bend your left leg and place your foot flat on the floor so that it is in front of you.

WATCHPOINTS

- Ensure this is not a continuous movement — remember to hold

- Don't let your leg touch the floor in between lifts

- To stop yourself rolling back, push your hips forward

3

Slowly raise your right leg off the floor (you will be able to go higher as you get stronger). Try to keep your leg straight and the toes flexed. Hold for a count of 2, then lower. Aim to do 16 lifts, then repeat on the other side.

Roll-ups

Tightening the oblique muscles of the waist, this exercise also tones your stomach. You may only manage 8 repetitions at first, but should be able to work up to 25 with a little practice.

Lie on your back with your knees bent, feet flat on the floor and hands down by your sides, palms facing up. Pull your stomach muscles towards your spine.

Curl your shoulders and head up and forward, keeping the lower part of your back on the floor.

Place your left hand beside your head with the elbow pointing towards your left knee. Lift your right arm off the floor, palm uppermost, keeping your arm low to begin with. As you lift the hand higher towards the knee you will feel your muscles tighten even more at the waist.

WATCHPOINTS

- Keep your lower back flat against the floor and tip your pelvis upward

- Breathe out on the way forwards and in on the way back

- Take each movement slowly and focus on the muscles you are working

4

Roll forwards and up as far as you can, keeping your chin pressed down to your chest, then lower back down to the starting position, but keep your shoulders just off the floor. Without pausing, repeat on the other side.

Bicycle abs

This exercise strengthens the rectus abdominus – the major muscles of the lower stomach. It also helps the external and internal oblique muscles, along with the hip flexors.

1

Lying on your back, bend both knees to 90 degrees. Place your hands on each side of your head.

2

Lift your head and shoulders off the mat.

3

Rotate your legs as if pedalling a bicycle, and move your torso from side to side as you push each elbow to the opposite knee.

WATCHPOINTS

- Make sure there is no stress on your neck

- Breathe out each time your knee comes in to your chest

- Keep your shoulders and head lifted off the floor throughout the exercise

Variation

Try keeping your legs straight as you move them out of each lift.

Crunches

- **REPS 10**
- **SETS 1–3**

Working on the major stomach muscles, including the external and internal obliques, this exercise will tone and tighten both the front and sides of your stomach.

1

Lie on your back with your knees bent and hip-width apart, feet flat on the floor. Place your hands on each side of your head.

2

Tighten your stomach muscles and lift your shoulders off the floor, exhaling as you do so. Keep your chin lifted. Hold for a count of 2. Inhale and lower slowly back down, but do not allow your shoulders to touch the floor.

WATCHPOINTS

- The effectiveness of this exercise depends on technique – keep it slow and controlled

- Don't pull on your neck or allow your back to arch

- Make sure both shoulders come off the floor and remain off throughout the exercise

Variation

For a more challenging version of this exercise, continue to curl upwards until your shoulders and upper back are lifted off the floor. Hold for a count of 2. Inhale and lower slowly back down, but do not allow your shoulders to touch the floor.

Scissors

This exercise tones the stomach and strengthens the legs, especially the quadriceps muscles and hip flexors. You may only manage a few scissors at first, but this will soon improve.

1

Lying on your back, rest back on your elbows with your hands flat on the floor and fingers pointing towards your bottom. Lean back slightly so your body is at 45 degrees to the floor. Bend your knees and draw them up to your chest.

2

Extend your legs so they are at 45 degrees to the floor. Pull your stomach muscles in and down.

WATCHPOINTS

- Don't allow your feet or legs to touch the floor

- There should be no strain through your back

- Keep your stomach tight with the muscles pulled down

3

Cross your right leg over your left and then your left leg over your right, moving them in a scissor action.

4

Scissor your legs up and down, taking them as high and as low as you can.

The plank

• REPS 2
• SETS 1–3

This exercise is great for strengthening your back, abdomen and shoulders. It works specifically on the transverse abdominus, the deepest abdominal muscle, to make your waist smaller.

WATCHPOINTS

- Maintain your body in a straight line from head to heels

- Keep your hips lifted and your stomach pulled up towards your spine

- Remember to breathe normally as you exercise

Lie face down with your elbows bent at 90 degrees under your shoulders and your palms and forearms flat on the floor. Push up from the floor, resting on your toes and elbows. Keeping your hips and back in a straight line, pull in your stomach and hold for a count of 20.

Variation

To increase the intensity of this exercise, lift your left leg straight out behind you and hold. Lower to the original position, then lift your right leg and hold as before.

Side bridge

This exercise targets the abdominals and the external and internal oblique muscles, working your waist and stomach. The longer you hold the lift, the more tension you place on the abdominals.

WATCHPOINTS

- Pull in your stomach muscles as you lift and keep them tight until you lower back down

- Keep your body in a straight line from shoulders to heels

- Don't let your hips drop

1

Lie on your right side with your body in a straight line and your left leg resting on your right. Rest on your right arm with the elbow bent.

2

Lift your pelvis off the floor, supporting your weight on your right forearm and feet. Your left arm rests on your left leg. Hold for a count of 10, then lower back down. Repeat 5-10 times on each side.

Reverse curls

This exercise will tone and strengthen the major stomach muscles including the rectus abdominus, and the hip flexors. You may find this a challenging exercise to begin with, but as your muscles strengthen you will be able to do more repetitions.

1

Lie on your back with your knees bent and your feet flat on the floor. Place your arms on each side of your body, resting on the floor. Bend your knees and lift your legs.

2

As you tighten your abdominal and stomach muscles, curl your pelvis and legs towards your ribcage, lifting your buttocks off the floor. Keep your legs at 90 degrees to your body. Exhale as you curl up and inhale as you lower back down.

WATCHPOINTS

- Slow, small, controlled movements are required to push your pelvis and lower back off the floor

- If you find this exercise difficult, cross your legs at the ankles

- Don't perform this exercise if you have lower back pain

Variation

To make this exercise more difficult, place your hands on each side of your head and lift your head, neck and shoulders off the floor at the same time as you lift your buttocks.

Tummy tighteners

- **REPS 10–20**
- **SETS 1–3**

Great for tightening the lower abdominal muscles, the hip flexors and the quadriceps muscles of the thighs, this exercise also strengthens the back's erector spinae and stabilizer muscles.

1

Sit with your knees bent, feet flat on the floor and hands resting on the floor on each side of your body.

2

Lean back slightly from the hips and lift both legs off the floor, keeping your knees slightly bent and toes pointing down.

WATCHPOINTS

- Keep your chin lifted

- There should be no strain through your neck

- Keep your stomach muscles pulled in and down

3

Release your arms, stretching them out in front of you, palms facing up. Hold for a count of 4, then lower back down to the starting position.

Variation

To increase the intensity of this exercise, straighten your legs and hold.

Oblique crunch

This exercise works the oblique muscles that run down the sides and front of your stomach as well as the upper abdominals. It is often used to target the 'love handles' at the sides of the waist.

1 Lie on your back with your knees bent and your left hand at the side of your head. Your right arm and hand rest on the floor. Cross your right leg over your left knee.

2 Lift your shoulder blades off the floor, supporting your head with your left hand.

WATCHPOINTS

- Don't thrust your head forward

- Don't pull on the back of your neck with your hands.

- Make sure you use your stomach muscles and not momentum to move

3

Curl your left upper body diagonally across towards your right knee and press your knee away from you. Repeat 10-20 times before changing sides, crossing your left leg over your right knee and lifting your right shoulder.

Double oblique crunch

Although this movement is very similar to the oblique crunch and works the same sets of muscles, it will also strengthen your back muscles and hip flexors.

- **REPS 10–20**
- **SETS 1–3**

1

Lie on your back with your knees bent, your legs held in the air and your hands on each side of your head.

2

Lift both shoulders up from the floor.

WATCHPOINTS

- Don't pull on your head or neck

- Keep your chin lifted as you crunch your knees in

- Make sure you are breathing correctly

3

Curl your legs and pelvis towards your ribcage, simultaneously curling your shoulders forwards. Exhale as you crunch your knees towards your left shoulder. Inhale as you lower back to the starting position. Repeat, bringing your knees in towards your right shoulder. Continue alternating left and right for 10–20 repetitions.

Heel touch

- REPS 10–20
- SETS 1–3

This is another great exercise for working the transverse muscle, the deepest of the stomach muscles and the one that supports the pelvis and lower back. It will help to flatten your stomach.

WATCHPOINTS

- Perform this exercise slowly – it does require good control to maximize its effectiveness

- If you need to make this exercise easier to begin with, bend your leg more and lower it to the floor closer to your buttocks

- Take care not to arch your back during this exercise

1

Lie on your back with your knees bent and feet flat on the floor. Place your hands flat on the floor beside your body. Lift your knees until your thighs are at 90 degrees to the floor.

2

Slowly lower your right leg, keeping your knee bent, and drop your heel to the floor.

3

Lift your right leg back up to your chest. Your left leg remains lifted. Bring your right knee back, next to your left knee. Repeat with your left leg.

Extended leg climb

- **REPS 5–10**
- **SETS 1–3**

This strong exercise challenges the abdominal muscles, including the rectus abdominus, the obliques and the hip flexors. Remember to pull your stomach muscles back and down towards your spine.

WATCHPOINTS

- Keep your elbows soft
- Don't swing your arms to reach forward
- Make sure you are breathing correctly

1

Lie on your back and lift your legs straight up above your hips. Keep your knees slightly bent. Place your hands on your shins while keeping your head and shoulders on the floor.

2

Raise your shoulders off the floor and at the same time move your arms up your shins, then lower back down. Exhale as you lift up and inhale as you lower.

Variation

For a more challenging version of this exercise, move your arms all the way up your shins and straighten your legs with each lift.

Groin stretch

• **REPS 1**
• **SETS 1**

This cool-down movement aids flexibility by stretching your groin area, the hip flexors including the psoas muscle and the adductor muscles of your inner thighs.

WATCHPOINTS

- **Stretch gently, taking care not to bounce**

- **Push your chest forward, not down, as this keeps your spine long**

1

Sit on the floor and put the soles of your feet together. Allow your knees to drop down. Place your hands on top of your feet or around your ankles and your elbows on the insides of your knees.

2

Lean forwards from the hips, flattening your back and pressing your knees gently down towards the floor.

Inner thigh stretch

This stretch will run from your groin, through your hip flexors including the psoas muscle, to the adductor muscles on the inside of your thighs.

WATCHPOINTS

1 2 3 4 5 6 7 8 9 10 11 12 13

• **Keep your upper body straight**

• **Make sure your heels are in a straight line before you begin**

Stand with your feet wide apart. Bend your right knee and take your body weight over to the right. Place both hands on your right thigh. Keep your left leg extended. Hold for a count of 10. Return to the starting position, then repeat to the left side.

Spinal twist

> • **REPS 1**
> • **SETS 1**

This stretch works your waist and lengthens your spine. It also stretches the hip flexors and the gluteal muscles of your buttocks, and improves posture.

1

Sit with your legs straight out in front of you. Place your hands flat on the floor on each side of your body. Cross your right leg over your left, bending your right knee and placing your right foot flat on the floor.

2

Place your left arm around your right knee so that your fingers and forearm rest on your outer right thigh. Using your left hand, bend your right leg and draw it towards the left side of your body.

WATCHPOINTS

- Keep your spine long and your shoulders relaxed and pulled down

- Exhale as you twist

- Keep your arm wrapped closely around your knee as you hug it to your chest

3

Curl your lower left leg around the right side of your body. Your left heel should be close to your right buttock. Turn your head and look over your right shoulder. Hold for a count of 5. Return to the starting position and repeat to the other side.

Pose of the child

This is a relaxation exercise as well as a stretch. You will feel the stretch through the spinal muscles, easing tension in your back, thighs and hips.

1

Kneel and sit back on your heels. Open your knees wide and lift both arms straight up to the ceiling.

2

Lower your chest and arms to the floor, with your buttocks remaining on your heels. Stretch forwards and hold for a count of 10. Lift your arms back up towards the ceiling, raising your chest to the starting position.

WATCHPOINTS

- Do not perform this exercise if you have any knee problems. However, the exercise can be used to relieve back pain.

- Breathe in and out gently as you remain in the lowered position.

- Inhale as you come back up to a sitting position.

1

Variation

Some people may be more comfortable using a towel to sit on during this stretch. Kneel as before, inserting a rolled-up towel behind your knees.

2

An easier variation is to stretch out your arms behind you as you lower your chest to the floor, holding for a count of 5.

Index

Acknowledgements

AUTHOR ACKNOWLEDGEMENTS

I would like to thank Jane and her team at Hamlyn.
Also, my sons, Alex and Harrison, Mum and Dad for their
continued support, Fiona for her culinary expertise and,
of course, Mark, for his inspiration.

PUBLISHER ACKNOWLEDGEMENTS

Executive editor Jane McIntosh
Editor Fiona Robertson
Executive art editor Karen Sawyer
Designer Martin Topping
Senior production controller Manjit Sihra
Picture library Sophie Delpech
Picture research Aruna Mathur

PICTURE ACKNOWLEDGEMENTS

Special Photography © **Octopus Publishing Group
Limited**/Mike Prior.

Alamy 36. **Corbis UK Limited**/LWA-Dann Tardif 13;
/George Shelley 8. **Getty Images** 21; /Brooke Fasani 6;
/Deborah Jaffe 9. **Octopus Publishing Group Limited**/
Frank Adam 14 centre left, 14 bottom right, 18 left, 34, 52,
68; /Stephen Conroy 33, 35, 37, 43, 47, 49, 62, 63, 64, 65;
/Jeremy Hopley 40; /David Jordan 17 bottom; /Sandra
Lane 14 top left, 44; /William Lingwood 14 centre right,
15, 28, 30, 46, 48, 66; /Peter Myers 17 top; /Sean Myers
14 bottom left; /Ian O'Leary 19; /Lis Parsons 29, 31, 39, 41,
45, 51, 53, 55, 57, 58, 59, 61, 67, 69; /Peter Pugh-Cook 75
bottom; /William Reavell 16, 32, 42; /Gareth Sambidge 18
right, 27, 50, 56; /Simon Smith 14 top right; /Ian Wallace
38, 54, 60. **Photolibrary** 74.